Women's Vulnerability to HIV/AIDS

Women's Vulnerability to HIV/AIDS

S.K. Singh
K.C. Das
H. Lhungdim

RAWAT PUBLICATIONS
Jaipur • New Delhi • Bangalore • Hyderabad • Guwahati • Kolkata

ISBN 978-81-316-0621-6

Published by
Prem Rawat for **Rawat Publications**
Satyam Apts, Sector 3, Jawahar Nagar, Jaipur 302 004 (India)
Phone: 0141 265 1748 / 7006 Fax: 0141 265 1748
E-mail: info@rawatbooks.com
Website: www.rawatbooks.com

New Delhi Office
4858/24, Ansari Road, Daryaganj, New Delhi 110 002
Phone: 011 2326 3290

Also at *Bangalore, Hyderabad, Guwahati* and *Kolkata*

Typeset by Rawat Computers, Jaipur
Printed at Chaman Enterprises, New Delhi

Contents

Preface

This book is an outcome of lessons learnt from an intervention, namely, 'Coordinated HIV/AIDS Response through Capacity Building and Awareness (CHARCA)' implemented by joint UN agencies in India under the leadership of UNAIDS, with the main objective to address young women's vulnerability to HIV/AIDS in India. The CHARCA baseline and endline surveys were conducted in five project districts, namely, Aizawl, Bellary, Guntur, Kanpur and Kishanganj, to assess the impact of CHARCA intervention programmes. The intervention was initiated in 2004 with the main objective of reducing young women's (age 13–24) vulnerability to STI/HIV. With evidence indicating that the risk of contracting HIV is much greater among young women due to the interplay of biological, economic and socio-cultural factors, the need to empower women along with providing a sound support system was realized. Accordingly, the intervention programmes were designed using a number of innovative approaches, targeting audience with specific messages to strengthen their knowledge and awareness about various preventive practices and behaviour change. Strategies adopted included creating legions of peer educators to facilitate awareness, capacity building, mobilization of local women groups and other organizations in supporting women to reduce their vulnerability with a rights-based approach.

The intervention programmes were implemented based on five CHARCA pillars, and the survey clearly brings out the impact of intervention in all the districts. The CHARCA intervention has succeeded in providing a framework for effective intervention to reduce vulnerability among young women in the five areas that are varied in terms of socio-economic as well as risk factors. The International Institute for Population Sciences (IIPS) undertook the task of conducting the baseline as well as endline surveys in the five districts. In this regard, we are thankful to Mr Alankar Malviya, the National Project Coordinator, CHARCA and other staff members at the CHARCA Secretariat, particularly Mr Upahar Pramanik, for their kind cooperation and support at different stages of the project. We also express our sincere gratitude to Professor (Late) P.N. Mari Bhat, the then Director, IIPS, for his encouragement and invaluable inputs at different stages of the project.

We also thank the coordinators of CHARCA District Management Units in each of the five districts for their kind cooperation and support during the fieldwork and to all our research team at IIPS, particularly Mr Suvakant Swain, Ms Amenla Nuken, and others who took up the strenuous task of fieldwork in different districts as well as data processing. We also express our gratitude to the language editor for editing the book. Finally, we express our sincere gratitude to all the respondents in the five districts for sparing their valuable time in providing necessary information.

S.K. Singh
K.C. Das
H. Lhungdim

List of Tables

List of Figures

Abbreviations

AIDS	Acquired Immune Deficiency Syndrome
ANC	Antenatal Care
ANM	Auxiliary Nurse Midwife
APMO	Assistant Para Medical Officer
ARO	Assistant Research Officer
ART	Antiretroviral Therapy
BL	Baseline
CBO	Community Based Organization
CHARCA	Co-ordinated HIV/AIDS Response through Capacity Building and Awareness
CHC	Community Health Centre
CRDS	Community Rural Development Society
CSW	Commercial Sex Worker
DM&HO	District Medical and Health Officer
DPMO	Deputy Para Medical Officer
DRDA	District Rural Development Authority
DSA	District Situational Assessment
DSP	District Strategic Plan
EL	Endline
FGD	Focus Group Discussion
FHAC	Family Health Awareness Campaign
GGH	Government General Hospital

GOI	Government of India
HIV	Human Immunodeficiency Virus
IIPS	International Institute for Population Sciences
IRDP	Integrated Rural Development Programme
IVDU	Intravenous Drug Users
KI	Key Informant
MDO	Mandal Development Officer
MPHA (F)	Multipurpose Health Worker (Female)/ANM
MPHA (M)	Multipurpose Health Worker (Male)
MPTC	Mandal Praja Tribunal Committee
MSM	Men having Sex with Men
NACO	National AIDS Control Organization
NGO	Non Governmental Organization
OBG	Obstetrics and Gynaecology
PD	Project Director
PHC	Primary Health Centre
PLWHA	Person Living with HIV/AIDS
PMO	Para Medical Officer
PMP	Private Medical Practitioner
PRD	Panchayat Raj Department
RC	Research Coordinator
RCH	Reproductive and Child Health
RI	Research Investigators
RMP	Rural Medical Practitioner/PMP
RO	Research Officer
RSC	Research Sub-Committee
RTI	Reproductive Tract Infection
SEEDS	Social Education and Economic Development Society
SC	Sub-Centre
STD	Sexually Transmitted Disease
STI	Sexually Transmitted Infection
UN	United Nations
UPHC	Upgraded Primary Health Centre
VCT	Voluntary Counselling and Testing
VCTC	Voluntary Counselling and Testing Centre

1

Introduction

Background and objectives

Over the years, there is growing evidence that the HIV epidemic in India is not restricted only to high-risk population but has emerged as a generalized epidemic at least in six high HIV prevalence states as well as in some selected pockets of moderate and low prevalence states. The new infections over a period of time have been marked by increasing female-male ratios and concentration among adolescents and youth. Therefore, the current scenario of the epidemic demands a concerted effort for prevention and control, which should primarily be designed in view of the risk factors associated with the vulnerability of the rural women in the country. The most recent round of Sentinel Surveillance, conducted through a network of more than seven hundred sites spread across the country, has shown that the prevalence of HIV has crossed one per cent level among pregnant women at least in the urban areas of seven states. There has been no systematic effort made to estimate the same among rural women, who are at a greater risk due to transmission of infection by a bridge population, from high risk commercial sex workers to low risk women population. However, there is a growing concern about the increasing incidence of RTIs/STDs/HIV among rural women and the psycho-social implications in the context of overall reproductive health of rural women. It is against this background that the CHARCA (Coordinated HIV/AIDS Response through Capacity Building and Awareness) efforts to enhance the extent of awareness and knowledge about STDs/HIV with development of community level support systems and an enabling environment (through multiple agencies) are found timely and need-based.

It is worth mentioning that the CHARCA intervention is expected to have a profound impact at targeting primarily young adults, preferably below 25 years of age. It is also expected to have a long-lasting and sustainable impact, as adolescence and early adulthood are distinct and dynamic phases of development in the life of an individual. This stage is characterized by spurts of physical, mental, emotional and social development. It is the time when influences outside the family assume greater significance. Adolescents find themselves facing new opportunities and challenges. It is also a formative stage in terms of sexual and reproductive maturity. Therefore, programmes and activities under the CHARCA intervention are extremely important for behavioural changes among adolescents and youth, which is likely to curb the pace of the HIV epidemic.

Traditional societies did not consider it necessary for adolescents to have information about sex prior to marriage believing that sexual activity occurs only within the wedlock. However, with modernization and the influence of mass media, the socio-cultural milieu has changed significantly, resulting in changes in values and norms related to sex and sexual behaviour. Adolescents are now often tempted to have sex before marriage. On the other hand, a considerable proportion of recently married women in India face coercive sex as they have limited choice to exercise during early marital sexual experiences. This may be primarily due to limited spousal intimacy in the context of desire for sex, which in turn results in restricted decisions regarding their own sexuality. Hence, their sexual behaviour depends primarily on their husband's/partner's desire for sex and behaviour.

In view of the above dimensions of risk behaviour among adolescents and early adults (below 25 years), irrespective of their marital status and need for a concerted effort, especially among rural adolescents, CHARCA intervention has been implemented to reduce the vulnerability of women, particularly young women (13–24 years), from HIV infection in six selected districts in India. The CHARCA project is a coordinated effort of the various UN agencies like UNDP, UNODC, UNIFEM, UNICEF, UNESCO, UNFPA, ILO, WHO and UNAIDS and aims to empower women to protect themselves against STI/HIV infections using a rights-based holistic approach. The project recognizes the fact that women, given their overall low and marginal status in society, are at great risk of acquiring HIV. The essential elements of the CHARCA programme are:

- to provide information related to sexually transmitted infections and rights issues;
- to improve accessibility to quality services;
- to build capacity and supporting network by providing a conducive environment that will empower women to protect themselves against STI/HIV; and
- to assert their rights effectively.

As part of the CHARCA evaluation plan, the International Institute for Population Sciences (IIPS), at the request of United Nations Development Programme (contract-2004–117 dated 7 June 2004), undertook the task of conducting a baseline survey in five districts, namely, Aizawl, Bellary, Guntur, Kanpur and Kishanganj. The main objective of the survey was to generate basic information among young women in order to strengthen capacity building activities and to develop appropriate programmes besides collecting information on various indicators of programme monitoring. The specific objectives of the CHARCA baseline survey were:

1. to examine knowledge, attitude, behaviour and practices related to STDs/HIV among rural women in the age group 13–25 years in five selected districts identified for CHARCA intervention in five different states;
2. to get qualitative insights about the attitudes of the target population in relation to collective action at community levels; and
3. to explore the problems and prospects of building local capacity, for example, local leadership and support networks to take up the issues of young women at community level, and developing sound referral systems for the reproductive and sexual health needs of adolescents.

After three years of community-based intervention through multiple approaches across five districts, this study has been conducted to assess the effectiveness of different components of CHARCA intervention and its impact in terms of five core issues addressed through different sets of programmes and activities, namely, awareness, capacity building, improved services, support system and enabling environment. The specific objectives of the CHARCA endline survey are:

- to have a comparative analysis with the baseline KABP survey in order to measure the changes in terms of knowledge, attitudes, behaviour and practices with respect to women's vulnerability to STI and HIV among CHARCA sub-populations in five CHARCA districts, and

- to evaluate the process adopted by CHARCA intervention in terms of engaging different stakeholders in collective action at the state, district and community levels to reduce young women's vulnerability to HIV/AIDS.

Research design

The endline survey has been conducted by using a combination of quantitative and qualitative tools in each of the five districts by adopting a suitably developed research design to measure the impact of CHARCA intervention through estimated change in some tangible behavioural parameters. A brief description of the methodology adopted for the quantitative components is presented below:

Determination of sample size

Given below are some important behavioural indicators included in CHARCA, providing a base for computation of the sample size in endline survey in a CHARCA district:

1. Young women's knowledge of at least one location from where male condoms can be obtained.
2. Young women's perception of 'sex with only one partner' as a measure to prevent HIV/AIDS.
3. Young women perceiving 'condom use' as a protection from acquiring HIV/AIDS.
4. Women are at higher risk of contracting STI/HIV than men.
5. Young women perceiving that the decision on 'utilization of health facilities' should be taken jointly with husband/partner.
6. Young women who mentioned 'STI/RTI/HIV' as a topic of discussion in the CBO/NGO meetings in last twelve months.
7. HIV positive people should mix with other or should visit public places.
8. Proportion of young women who reported to have had sex first before 15 years of their age.
9. Young women who sought treatment in 'government hospitals' for STI during the last twelve months.
10. Young women who 'experienced any type of violence'.

Sample sizes to capture expected outcomes in some key behavioural indicators across different districts included in CHARCA intervention have been calculated on the basis of the following factors typically used in surveys with probability samples:

Table 1.1

Estimated sample size to capture expected change in proportion of young women reporting different behavioural parameters across CHARCA districts

Indicators	*Observed (P_1)*	*Expected (P_2)*	*P= (P_1+ P_2)/2*	*Design effect*	*Estimated # sample women*	*Approximate Number of HHs to get sample women*
Proportion of young women who reported to have had sex first before 15 years of their age	0.33	0.28	0.35	2	3,825	6,500
Young women who reported any STI during last twelve months	0.52	0.45	0.48	2.28	2,510	4,270
Young women knowing at least one location of getting male condom	0.43	0.53	0.48	2.36	1,270	2,160
Young women perceiving decision on 'utilization of health facilities' should be taken jointly with husband/partner	0.62	0.72	0.67	2.17	1,034	1,760
Women are at higher risk of contracting STI/HIV than men	0.49	0.6	0.55	2	885	1,505
Young women who mentioned knowledge about functioning of CBOs/NGOs in their locality	0.4	0.55	0.475	3.02	720	1,225
HIV positive people should not mix with other	0.51	0.45	0.48	2	3,000	5,100
Young women experienced any type of violence	0.17	0.1	0.135	2	1,030	1,750
Young women perceiving 'sex with only one partner' as a measure to prevent HIV/AIDS	0.66	0.75	0.71	2	1,100	1,870
Young women perceiving 'condom use' as a protection from acquiring HIV/AIDS	0.58	0.68	0.63	2	1,005	1,710

1. The observed value of the indicator in the baseline survey;
2. Expected magnitude of change which can be attributed to the programmatic response rather than due to fluctuation of sampling with the computed sample size;
3. Confidence level;
4. Statistical power; and
5. Design effect.

The following formula has been used to determine the sample size to capture expected change in different behavioural indicators included in the CHARCA intervention:

$$n = D\frac{[Z_{1-\alpha}\sqrt{2P(1-P)} + Z_{1-\beta}\sqrt{P_1(1-P_1)+P_2(1-P_2)}]^2}{(P_2-P_1)^2}$$

Where:

D = Design effect.

P_1 = the estimated proportion of the indicator at the time of CHARCA baseline survey conducted in July 2004.

P_2 = The expected proportion of the same indicator in March 2007, such that the quantity (P_2 - P_1) is the size of the magnitude of change desired to be detected through sample of size n.

P = $(P_1 + P_2)/2$

$Z_{1-\alpha}$ = The z-score corresponding to the probability with which it is desired to be able to conclude that an observed change of size (P_2 - P_1) would not have occurred by chance or due to fluctuation of sampling.

$Z_{1-\beta}$ = The z-score corresponding to the degree of confidence with which it is desired to be certain of detecting a change of size (P_2 - P_1) if one actually occurred.

It is evident from the above table that the estimated sample of young women aged 13–24 and the approximate number of households to be approached for getting the desired number (by considering age-sex composition of population) to detect the desired change in the above behavioural parameters varies from a minimum of 1,225 households to the maximum of 6,500 households in all the five districts. Therefore, the ideal sample size for CHARCA endline survey would be 3,825 young women who can be approached by selecting 6,500 households, i.e., 1,300 households per district. However, using the experience of the baseline survey it was decided to select 55 households per PSU and hence the sampling design used for the endline survey included 23

PSUs per district (as against 15 PSUs in the baseline survey). This has provided an opportunity to consider over 50 per cent of baseline PSUs as panel PSUs (only among rural PSUs) and 15 new PSUs have been randomly selected by adopting a two-stage design for rural PSUs and a three-stage design for urban PSUs as in the baseline survey.

Sampling design

Once the sample size and number of PSUs to be included in the study is determined for both rural and urban areas in a district, selection of sampling units, i.e., women in the age group 13–24 years (16 to 27 years in case of panel PSUs), has been carried out following a multi-stage random sampling procedure.

The rural sample was selected using a two-stage design, with selection of villages by probability proportional to size (PPS) after grouping them according to their distance from the district headquarters (less than 5 km, 5–10 km, and more than 10 km). At the second stage, selection of a fixed number of households was done using systematic sampling within each selected village after complete listing of households. However, in case of large villages with more than 400 households, the villages were divided into a minimum of three segments and two segments were randomly selected for complete house listing and selection of a fixed number of households.

In urban areas, a three-stage procedure was adopted. In the first stage, a ward was selected with PPS, followed by the selection of a cluster/section again by PPS. Lastly, a fixed number of households were selected from each cluster after comprehensive house listing. The process of segmentation of section/cluster was also used in the urban areas where size of the section or cluster was more than 500 households.

Further, the selection of the eligible men (males age 15–29) was done exclusively from those selected households where at least one eligible woman was recorded at the screening level. Thus, out of 55 selected households in a PSU, two types of households, namely, 'where neither a woman aged 13–24 years nor a male aged 15–29 years have been recorded' and 'households not having any target women but having at least one target male' were not considered in the survey. As a result, male interviews were conducted only in those households where the eligible men and women had been recorded through the screening preformed.

In case of panel PSUs, the research team made its best effort to interview the maximum number of women possible who were included in the baseline survey. Due to a gap of almost three years in the survey, there was very little chance of interviewing unmarried girls who had been interviewed in the baseline survey. Therefore, we developed a survey protocol to select all the eight panel PSUs among rural PSUs and to interview only married respondents who had been interviewed in the baseline survey.

Design for the qualitative study

A series of ethnographic research tools have been used in order to get comprehensive insights into the processes attuned with the second objective of the study, which is extremely useful in learning about strengths and weaknesses of CHARCA programmes and activities on the one hand and prioritizing issues for replication and upscaling of such programmes on the other. Given below is the sequence of implementing ethnographic tools with predefined roles and objectives consistent with the inputs in implementation of CHARCA efforts across different districts:

- *Listing of community-based resources for women:* As a part of assessment of the impact of CHARCA intervention, all the opportunities/institutions developed or strengthened as a part of the intervention, including the existing local resources such as CBOs, and other women's groups, etc., have been approached. It has been attempted to assess the process through which these institutions have addressed women-related issues, especially their capacity building. These interactions include information on organizational structure, frequency of meeting, roles, functions and responsibilities, especially in the context of women's issues.
- *Key informant interviews*: Community level stakeholders have been interviewed in order to get insights into the problems and prospects to activate CBOs and other women's groups in the context of women's issues including reproductive health problems and reproductive rights. Local political leaders, religious leaders, office bearers of women's organizations and other influential persons have also been interviewed as key informants in a village or an urban block with the help of a predefined check list.
- *Focus group discussion*: In view of certain limitations of social mapping providing positioning and placement of organizational

set-ups required to assess the impact of the programme, the endline survey has collected data on the functional efficacy of the programme more adequately and easily through focus group discussions (FGDs) among CHARCA sub-populations in addition to key informant interviews. However, in order to enhance in-depth understanding of the programme impact, FGDs among different groups like young women, young men, peer educators, PLWHA (persons living with HIV/AIDS), IVD users (intravenous drug users) have been conducted in each of five districts.

Quality check measures

In any community-based survey, strategies to ensure quality of information is vital for the validity and reliability of information. This study has adopted the following specific measures to ensure quality of information collected:

1. A comprehensive house listing in each selected PSU to minimize the arbitrariness in selection of households and target respondents.
2. Comprehensive training of investigators and field practices with special emphasis on qualitative techniques by first organizing training of trainers workshop at the institute jointly with CHARCA secretariat.
3. Developing standard survey protocols for the entire field operation starting from rapport building, house listing, selection of households, canvassing of screener to canvassing of individual level interviews in the households qualified for the individual level interviews.
4. Suitable sex composition of investigators (4 female and 2 male investigators) in order to ensure quality of responses from males as well as from females at different levels of survey.
5. Use of standard text to introduce the project across different districts and PSUs. It has also been beneficial in developing excellent rapport with community level stakeholders, heads of the selected households and respondents.
6. Qualitative research tools, viz., resource mapping, key informants interviews and FGDs have been canvassed by supervisors (RO and AROs) trained student of IIPS, who had undergone an advance course in research methodology as part of their Master's Course in Population Studies.
7. Two-stage monitoring and supervision of the field operations in order to ensure the quality of data by ROs and faculty co-coordinators.

8. Identification of local NGOs, and involvement of some of their selected staff in the training programme for the research investigators as a means to their capacity building.

Profiles of respondents

Information on socio-economic and demographic profile of the respondents was collected in all the five CHARCA districts. The information included in the endline survey throws light on the background of the respondents and is quite useful in effectively answering to some of the research questions formulated in the study. Table 1.2 presents the per cent distribution of female respondents aged 13–24 by some selected background characteristics collected both in the baseline (2004) and endline (2007) surveys. For getting insight into the age-wise variation of respondents across five CHARCA districts, the broad age group of 13–24 years has been classified into three age groups – 13–16 years, 17–20 years and 21–24 years – in order to maintain homogeneity in the age intervals. More than one-third of the respondents in each of the five districts belong to the age group 17–20 in both the surveys. Thus, there is no significant skewness in the age distribution across different districts in the endline as well as the baseline surveys. The distribution of respondents by marital status reveals that a considerably higher proportion of respondents (84%) in the baseline as well as the endline surveys in Aizawl are unmarried but the pattern remains by and large the same. The other three districts of Kishanganj, Bellary and Guntur have relatively a lower proportion of unmarried respondents. Thus, the existing variation in marital status may help in getting insight if there are considerable differences in perception and behaviours.

Educational attainment of the female is an important parameter in explaining the success of any programme. Looking at the variation of the educational attainment of the respondents, it is evident from Table 1.2 that more than 30 per cent of the illiterate women at both the periods are found in Kishanganj and Bellary, though it has declined marginally over the periods. While the proportion of such women in Guntur during baseline was 25 per cent where it has declined to 6 per cent and it was 9 per cent in Kanpur during the endline survey. On the other hand, almost all the respondents in Aizawl are educated. Data on husband's education reveals that only Kishanganj has higher (above 30%) proportion of illiteracy among husbands at both the periods. While in Bellary, though the proportion was 3 per cent during the baseline survey, it has increased to 45 per cent during the endline

Table 1.2

Profile of the female respondents in the five CHARCA districts (%)

Background characteristics	*Kanpur**	*Kishanganj*		*Bellary*		*Guntur*		*Aizawl*	
	EL	*BL*	*EL*	*BL*	*EL*	*BL*	*EL*	*BL*	*EL*
Age (completed years)									
13–16	**31.6**	35.7	**23.7**	28.8	**32.7**	28.2	**23.3**	29.1	**26.0**
17–20	**39.5**	32.7	**35.3**	41.9	**37.2**	43.5	**37.4**	40.2	**40.3**
21–24	**28.9**	31.4	**41.1**	29.3	**30.0**	28.2	**39.3**	30.8	**33.7**
Marital Status									
Married	**34.2**	42.5	**53.3**	58.2	**46.9**	53.8	**56.4**	17.8	**16.4**
Unmarried	**65.6**	57.5	**46.7**	41.8	**51.8**	46.2	**43.6**	82.2	**83.6**
Women's Education									
Illiterate	**9.3**	39.1	**36.6**	35.5	**30.2**	24.5	**6.2**	0.6	**0.2**
<5 years complete	**4.0**	22.4	**19.4**	10.7	**10.8**	5.3	**15.8**	3.6	**0.5**
5–7 years complete	**12.0**	19.1	**18.9**	22.3	**20.0**	26.9	**29.7**	21.3	**10.0**
8–9 years complete	**29.4**	10.2	**12.0**	15.0	**14.7**	9.8	**14.9**	34.7	**31.4**
10 and above	**45.3**	9.1	**13.1**	16.6	**24.3**	33.5	**33.3**	39.8	**57.9**
Husband's Education									
Illiterate	**7.1**	29.9	**34.3**	3.2	**45.2**	31.9	**10.7**	1.3	—
<5 years complete	**1.8**	17.5	**17.3**	10.0	**7.3**	5.0	**9.0**	3.9	—
5–7 years complete	**9.5**	18.6	**20.2**	24.2	**16.5**	24.4	**40.6**	22.1	**2.8**
8–9 years complete	**30.2**	16.4	**12.1**	17.9	**6.1**	7.1	**8.1**	31.2	**25.0**
10 and above	**51.5**	17.4	**16.1**	44.7	**25.0**	31.5	**31.6**	41.6	**72.2**
Membership in CBOs/NGOs									
Yes	**3.4**	1.1	**4.9**	4.5	**27.4**	14.6	**45.6**	57.1	**86.8**
No	**63.8**	98.9	**0.6**	95.5	**72.3**	85.4	**50.8**	42.9	**13.2**
Women's Occupation									
Homemaker	**93.7**	94.8	**94.3**	58.8	**59.9**	60.6	**79.6**	87.3	**92.7**
Working as Labourer/family farm	**4.9**	3.5	**3.5**	35.0	**34.5**	36.7	**19.4**	8.7	**5.0**
Salaried/paid job	**1.4**	1.7	**2.2**	6.1	**0.9**	2.8	**1.0**	4.0	**2.3**
Migratory Status of Husband									
Non-migrant	**82.5**	95.2	**95.2**	99.4	**59.2**	99.6	**76.1**	99.4	**89.8**
Migrant	**17.5**	4.8	**4.8**	0.6	**40.8**	0.4	**23.9**	0.6	**10.2**
Exposure to Mass Media									
Yes	**89.1**	77.4	**74.8**	90.0	**89.9**	83.9	**96.9**	99.4	**99.8**
No	**10.9**	22.6	**25.2**	10.0	**10.1**	16.1	**3.1**	0.6	**0.2**
Total Respondents	**494**	539	**465**	488	**556**	472	**417**	471	**439**

* Information from the baseline survey is not presented due to change in intervention after the baseline survey.

EL: endline, BL: baseline

period. In Guntur, it has declined from 32 per cent to 11 per cent, while in Kanpur it was 7 per cent in the endline survey.

Membership in community-based organizations (CBOs) or non-government organizations (NGOs) deserves special attention as it is likely to affect knowledge, attitude and behaviour with respect to different aspects of study subjects. This is a very important component of CHARCA intervention since it is meant to provide a support system to the young women and empower the community to reduce contextual determinants of women's vulnerability to STI/HIV. It is evident from Table 1.2 that the percentage of women having membership in CBOs/NGOs has increased in each of the five districts over the baseline survey. This may be due the programmes and activities of CHARCA resulting in more female becoming members of various CBOs/NGOs. Bellary, Guntur and Aizawl have recorded significant increase in the proportion of young women having CBOs/NGOs membership. On the other hand, Kishanganj has recorded only a marginal increase and the majority are still not members of any CBO/NGO.

The occupational status of the women shows that about nine-tenths of them in Aizawl, Kishanganj and Kanpur are engaged in homemaking profession, while the proportion of such women is comparatively lower in Bellary and Guntur. On the other hand, more than one-third of respondents in Bellary and one-fifth in Guntur are working as daily wage labourers. The distribution of young women by their main occupation across the CHARCA districts does not change significantly over the baseline except in Guntur, where there is a shift from working as labourer and working on family farm to homemaker.

The migratory status of the husbands has been attracting increased attention of the researchers and programme personnel, especially in view of its potential to increase women's vulnerability to STI/HIV infections. In the CHARCA baseline as well as endline surveys, women whose husbands were working away from home and visited them once or twice a month have been considered as wives of migrants. It is evident from Table 1.2 that nearly all the respondents at the time of baseline survey in Bellary, Guntur and Aizawl (except Kishanganj) had their husbands as non-migrants. However, the pattern has been reversed in the endline survey among the respondents.

The exposure of the population to various mass media is very important in creating awareness about different programmes. The data from the endline survey reveals that little over a quarter (25.2%) of the respondents in Kishanganj, 11 per cent in Kanpur, 10 per cent in Bellary and 3 per cent in Guntur are not exposed to any mass media.

Almost everybody in Aizawl is exposed to one or the other forms of mass media.

Table 1.3 presents the profile of male respondents in the CHARCA baseline as well as endline surveys. The age of the eligible male respondents (15–29), which has been considered for the interview, has been classified into two broad categories, namely, up to 20 years and more than 20 years. It is evident from the Table 1.3 that about two-fifths of the respondents from Kishanganj, Bellary and Guntur districts were below 20 years of age in the baseline survey. The proportion of male respondents below age 20 has decreased in all the districts barring Kanpur. The distribution of respondents by their marital status shows that the proportion of unmarried respondents has declined in the endline survey in comparison to the baseline survey.

Table 1.3

Profile of the male respondents in the five CHARCA districts (%)

Background characteristics	*Kanpur**	*Kishanganj*		*Bellary*		*Guntur*		*Aizawl*	
	EL	*BL*	*EL*	*BL*	*EL*	*BL*	*EL*	*BL*	*EL*
Age									
<=20 years	**47.2**	43.0	**37.5**	41.4	**38.8**	37.5	**32.7**	54.1	**47.8**
20+ years	**52.8**	57.0	**62.5**	58.6	**61.2**	62.5	**67.3**	45.9	**52.2**
Marital Status									
Unmarried	**60.9**	58.8	**54.3**	53.1	**56.5**	44.3	**38.3**	77.7	**19.0**
married	**39.1**	41.2	**45.7**	46.9	**43.5**	55.7	**61.7**	22.3	**81.0**
Education									
Illiterate	**0.9**	35.2	**31.4**	18.9	**26.8**	11.8	**0.0**	0.0	**0.0**
<5 years complete	**6.5**	23.9	**7.9**	13.8	**8.8**	5.3	**6.5**	4.1	**0.5**
5–7 years complete	**11.2**	13.7	**19.8**	14.6	**17.4**	26.5	**35.0**	15.6	**0.0**
8–9 years complete	**31.1**	14.8	**14.3**	14.6	**11.0**	8.6	**9.1**	37.2	**7.1**
10 and above	**50.3**	12.3	**26.5**	38.2	**36.0**	48.2	**48.7**	43.1	**92.4**
Membership in CBOs									
Yes	**2.5**	44.4	**37.3**	11.1	**11.8**	19.5	**41.4**	97.3	**92.4**
No	**97.5**	55.6	**62.7**	88.9	**88.2**	80.5	**58.6**	2.7	**6.5**
Total Respondents	**322**	291	**328**	256	**317**	264	**214**	220	**184**

* Information from the baseline survey is not presented due to change in intervention after the baseline survey

The educational attainment of respondents has an important bearing on their awareness and perceptions relating to different dimensions of core indicators of the CHARCA programmes and activities. About one-third of the respondents in Kishanganj were illiterate during both the periods of the survey. On the other hand, all the respondents in Aizawl were literate.

Regarding membership in CBOs/NGOs, more than 90 per cent of male respondents in Aizawl were members of CBOs/NGOs, followed by Guntur (41%) and Kishanganj (37%). While the proportion of such membership has declined in Kishanganj over the period of time, it registered a significant increase in Guntur during the inter-survey period.

Organization of chapters

This book has eight chapters including an executive summary. The current chapter introduces the survey.

Chapter 2 deals with different sources of knowledge about reproductive health issues among young women and men during the process of their growing up, i.e., proportion of young women reporting womenfolk, peers and friends as sources of knowledge about reproductive health issues during the process of growing up. It also discuses the knowledge of young women about any source of getting male condom, the incidence of menstrual problems during 12 months prior to the survey and treatment seeking, especially with focus on government health facilities.

Chapter 3 deals with knowledge and awareness of reproductive and sexual health including STI/HIV prevention. It is based on different indicators dealing with different dimensions of awareness, namely, women and men knowing that consistent use of condom during each sexual intercourse can protect them from STI/HIV infections, women having at least one misconception of HIV/AIDS transmission, different modes of preventing from STI/HIV transmission, HIV testing among young women and men, and knowledge of a source where one can get tested for his/her HIV status. Towards the end, people's attitudes towards HIV positive individuals have also been presented.

Chapter 4 presents information relating to capacity building of women in the context of their knowledge and skill to protect themselves from STI/HIV infections. It has been organized under two domains, namely, reproductive and sexual rights. Both the domains have been further classified with the help of core indicators included in the frame of CHARCA. Some of the important indicators analysed in this chapter are young women and men who perceive that the decision about the number of children should be taken jointly by husband and wife, young women and men who perceive that the decision about utilization of healthcare facilities should be taken jointly by husband and wife, young women and men who perceive that the husband should be accepted under any condition, even if he has extramarital relationships, and young women who do not have the ability to refuse sex when they do not want it.

Chapter 5 shows the incidence of violence against women in the CHARCA districts and relative changes over the baseline survey. Some of the selected indicators analysed in this chapter are membership in CBOs/NGOs, major issues discussed during meetings, women who have experienced violence, women who sought formal support system in case of violence and so on. Another important issue covered in this chapter is the type of support system in case of violence against women. A comparison of baseline and endline surveys on type of support system provides a clue to assess the efficacy and impact of CHARCA interventions in reducing violence against women.

Chapter 6 discusses the symptomatic prevalence of STIs among women and men across CHARCA districts, their treatment-seeking behaviour and perceived quality of STI services. These discussions are based on selected indicators revealing their potential for early diagnosis and treatment of STIs as a means of reducing women's vulnerability to STIs/HIV. Some of the core indicators analysed in this chapter are young women and men who have at least one symptom of STIs during the last 12 months, women and men by place of last treatment sought, and young women and men who reported the availability of at least three quality parameters at the place where service was last sought for STI infections.

Chapter 7 contains information pertaining to the functional efficacy of CHARCA intervention. It has been based on four scales developed after testing of reliability of statements showing people's perception on impact of CHARCA programmes and activities in enhancing awareness, capacity building of women, empowerment of women and improved services. Variations in the values of scales have been analysed by some selected socio-economic and demographic characteristics of respondents.

2

Knowledge of Reproductive and Sexual Health Issues in the Process of Growing up

Transitions from childhood to adolescence and early adulthood are distinct and dynamic phases of development in the life of an individual. This stage is characterized by spurts of physical, mental, emotional and social development. It is the time when influences outside the family assume greater significance and also a formative stage in terms of sexual and reproductive maturity (Singh et al., 2004). Therefore, sources of information on family life education, especially reproduction and reproductive health, are extremely important for perceptions and behaviour, which ultimately influence the health and well-being of youth of a nation. In countries like India, traditional societies did not consider it necessary for adolescents to have information about sex prior to marriage believing that sexual activity occurs only within the wedlock. However, with modernization and the influence of mass media, the socio-cultural milieu has changed significantly, resulting in changes in values and norms related to sex and sexual behaviour. Adolescents are now often tempted to have sex before marriage. On the other hand, a substantial proportion of recently married women in India face coercive sex as they have limited choice to exercise during early marital sexual experiences.

The phase of adolescence and early adulthood for boys (age 13–25 years), irrespective of their marital status, is marked by a strong desire to experiment largely influenced by friends and peer groups. During this stage of life, peer relations become more intense and adolescents start spending more time outside the home, escaping the companionship of the adult members of their families. The influence of mass media, friends and peer groups provokes them to experiment risky lifestyle activities resulting in increased prevalence of sexually transmitted diseases (STDs) including HIV/AIDS. Over a period, there is growing evidence of increasing concentration of STI and HIV among adolescents and youth.

Adolescents are particularly vulnerable to STDs, including HIV/AIDS, because of high-risk behaviour, little knowledge of preventive measures, greater biological susceptibility to infections and limited access to health facilities for treatment. Therefore, it is essential to develop a suitable strategy for providing comprehensive knowledge of reproductive health issues and effective behaviour change to both adolescents and youth in India.

CHARCA intervention has included a comprehensive awareness programme through a peer-based model in all the five districts and this chapter attempts to analyse the effectiveness of CHARCA intervention by examining the changes in sources of knowledge among young women and men. This chapter has been organized into three sections. The first section deals with the sources of knowledge among young women and men during the process of their growing up whereas awareness about different sources of getting male condoms have been presented in the second section. The third section presents the prevalence of menstrual health problems among women aged 13–24 in the 12 months prior to the baseline and endline surveys and their treatment-seeking behaviour.

Sources of information in the process of growing up

The Government of India has been using mass media extensively, especially electronic media, to increase awareness of family life issues among adolescents so that they can have comprehensive knowledge of reproductive health issues. The CHARCA intervention also had a mandate to encourage parents, school teachers and health professional to discus reproductive health issues to children during the process of their growing up. In the baseline as well as in the endline surveys, young women and men were asked about the main source of their information on reproductive health issues, especially changes in their body at puberty including menstruation and the results are presented in Tables 2.1 and 2.2.

Table 2.1

Source of information for young women during the process of growing up (up to age 15) in the five CHARCA districts (%)

Source of information	*Kanpur**	*Kishanganj*		*Bellary*		*Guntur*		*Aizawl*	
	EL	*BL*	*EL*	*BL*	*EL*	*BL*	*EL*	*BL*	*EL*
Womenfolk†	88.7	97.6	95.3	96.1	68.7	99.4	79.9	81.3	72.2
Peers/friends	32.0	81.0	37.6	77.0	30.9	92.6	58.3	55.5	54.4
Schools/teachers	7.0	3.7	0.6	23.2	16.7	21.7	6.5	12.4	30.1
Media‡	25.5	54.2	6.5	61.9	24.8	71.2	8.6	30.6	59.7
Health service providers	5.3	1.3	0.2	2.9	13.1	3.2	7.0	2.8	4.6
Total respondents	494	538	465	487	556	472	417	471	439

*Information from the baseline survey is not presented due to change in intervention after the baseline survey.

† Womenfolk means mother/sister/sister-in-law.

‡ Media include newspapers/magazines/ books/television.

Table 2.1 presents the sources of information during the process of growing up for young women in different districts over the project periods. In each of the five districts womenfolk have been reported as the main sources of information for young women during their process of growing up, followed by peers/friends. In the endline survey, womenfolk as the main source of information range from a minimum of 69 per cent in Bellary to the maximum of 95 per cent in Kishanganj. The proportion who mentioned peers/friends ranges from 32 per cent in Kanpur to 58 per cent in Guntur. Though mentioned by a small proportion of young women, health service providers as a source of information about family life education shows an increase over the years. On average, more than 3 per cent women mentioned health service providers as a source of information during the process of their growing up.

Another equally important issue is the contribution of schools and teachers in imparting information on family life education to adolescents during the process of their growing up. Both these contributions, i.e., increasing role of health providers and schools/teachers in imparting information pertaining to family life education can be attributed to CHARCA programmes and activities. These findings are also supported by insights into these processes through KIs (key informants) and FGDs (focus group discussions).

'... the programmes like 'nukkad natak' have influenced the life of the villagers and made them especially women much informed and aware about HIV/AIDS and other related issues ...'

—Woman KI, Kanpur

'... the activities and programmes conveying the messages about hygiene, healthcare, AIDS, women rights and other women issues have generated concern on several vital matters related to well-being among the women and empowered them to fight for their rights of well-being ...'

—Man KI, Aizawl

'... street plays followed by flip chart shows are very effective, the information is presented in an interesting way for easy understanding of the whole issue of health, lifestyle and self-esteem ... the women have become aware about HIV/AIDS and the modes and ways of its transmission and prevention ...'

—Peer FGD, Kanpur

'... the messages are given with interesting illustrations so that people can relate them with their own life through this programme. It gives them ready-made examples to think upon their own way and how they are behaving in different situations and how they should behave to protect their rights and prestige ...'

—Man KI, Bellary

'... women who participate in the programmes and activities always come back and ask their doubts on different health issues; sometimes they even ask beyond the programme message which shows their growing interest in learning and knowing healthy life skill'.

—Peer FGD, Kishanganj

The qualitative insights reveal the effectiveness of the programme designed and implemented to enhance the awareness among young women across the five CHARCA districts. Culture sensitivity in conveying the message regarding awareness, correct knowledge and behavioural change motivation have been found to be largely accepted and appreciated by the communities. Such programmes have successfully reflected the day-to-day life issues of the women and men in the community and have motivated them to monitor their own behaviour and rights at different levels.

Table 2.2

Source of information for men during the process of growingup (up to age 15) in the five CHARCA districts (%)

Source of information (up to age 15)	*Kanpur**	*Kishanganj*		*Bellary*		*Guntur*		*Aizawl*	
	EL	*BL*	*EL*	*BL*	*EL*	*BL*	*EL*	*BL*	*EL*
Friends/peers	89.8	99.0	39.6	92.2	52.7	94.7	66.3	85.7	85.3
Parents/family	25.2	28.3	9.5	5.5	38.8	0.8	10.3	25.1	14.1
Teachers/schools	16.5	7.9	4.9	15.2	24.3	5.7	32.7	42.1	55.4
Books/magazines/posters/ Television/movies	81.1	92.1	10.1	95.3	36.0	95.8	53.7	80.9	91.8

* Information from the baseline survey is not presented due to change in intervention after the baseline survey.

Young men were also asked about the main source of information during the process of their growing up. A majority of them men mentioned two main sources of information, namely, friends/peers and electronic and print media including books/magazines/posters/television/movies in the baseline as well as the endline surveys. Though parents/family and teachers/schools are the least mentioned sources of information across the five CHARCA districts, their contribution in imparting knowledge on these issues has increased over the baseline survey.

The contribution of schools/teachers in imparting knowledge to young boys during the process of their growing up is consistent with the pattern emerging in case of sources of information among young girls. In addition, the credit to break the culture of silence between parents and their children should be given to peer educators of CHARCA who have recently contributed in enhancing community awareness.

Knowledge about sources of getting male condom

In the HIV prevention programme, correct and consistent use of condom has been given top priority along with a comprehensive knowledge of preventive practices. However, there is increasing evidence of unprotected sexual intercourse even after awareness. It is against this backdrop that the CHARCA has addressed safe sexual practices within a rights perspective. In fact, attitudes towards a woman's right to negotiate sex with her husband are likely to be influenced by a number of social, cultural and traditional norms and values

'... the programme at railway station that says about the condom use importance is really interesting, it clearly gives a message that those who don't accept condom use, they always put themselves at risk of getting STIs and even AIDS ...'

—Man FGD, Guntur

'... the dramas and charts are revealing the knowledge and information which were not known before or nobody was comfortable to pass this information to younger generation; at the same time, its important to have this knowledge too. It is a matter of relief that our boys are also interested to learn ...'

—Woman KI, Aizawl

'... these issues related to taking care of general health, sexual health, dealing with women, etc., are important and in family we can't discuss. Many times friends and seniors are the main source of giving ideas and notions regarding these issues but they also have their own perceptions and misconceptions. The programmes are very beneficial to get the correct knowledge in this situation ...'

—Man FGD, Kanpur

'... I like the plays and the way they make the knowledge entertaining. It attracts more people to watch and give the messages. If you call people just to attend meetings of any informative session, they may not turn up in this number ...'

—Man KI, Bellary

'... they remember the characters of the plays and ask us on certain issues referring to some situation of the plays and other programmes ... it surely implies the impact of the programme on the young minds ... in a rural set-up where most of the modern ways of entertainment are not available to young people, the plays and other dramatically representations are much popular ...'

—Peer FGD, Kishanganj

prevailing in both traditional and transitional societies. Therefore, the indicator used by CHARCA is the proportion of young women who are aware of different sources of getting male condom. Accordingly, the issue has been explored in both baseline and endline surveys and the results are presented in Tables 2.3 and 2.4.

Young women in the study population were asked whether or not they are aware about any location or place where they could get male condoms. Young women in Aizawl (91%) and Guntur (84%) are more likely to know about this compared to those in other CHARCA districts. The proportion of such women is the lowest in Kishanganj (45%). There is a definite impact of CHARCA programmes and activities in enhancing awareness about sources of getting male condoms in all the four districts except Kishanganj (Kanpur has been omitted from this analysis due to change in intervention area). The increase in the proportion of young women knowing at least one location to get male condom is the highest in Guntur (from 20% to 84%), followed by Bellary (from 11% to 67%) and Aizawl (42% to 91%).

Table 2.3

Percentage of women who are aware of different locations to get male condoms in the five CHARCA districts

	*Kanpur**	*Kishanganj*		*Bellary*		*Guntur*		*Aizawl*	
	EL	*BL*	*EL*	*BL*	*EL*	*BL*	*EL*	*BL*	*EL*
Medical stores	61.5	52.5	34.2	9.6	53.4	14.4	81.8	21	82.5
Health personnel	15.2	2.8	31.6	11.1	47.3	16.7	60.2	12.8	40.3
NGOs/CBOs	11.5	0.0	0.2	2.7	22.1	10.8	15.8	27	41.5
Shops	27.3	7.0	26.2	4.6	22.3	12.8	37.9	3.4	2.5
Knowing at least one location	62.6	54	44.9	11.5	66.6	19.7	84.2	41.8	90.9
Total Women	494	538	465	475	556	471	417	468	439

* Information from the baseline survey is not presented due to change in intervention after the baseline survey.

Women reported different locations to get male condoms and these vary from district to district (Figure 2.1). In districts such as Guntur and Aizawl young women mentioned at least two or three locations for getting condoms. But in other districts like Kanpur, Kishanganj and Bellary, young women are generally less likely to know more locations to get male condoms. The most frequently reported location for getting male condoms is the medical store, ranging from 34 per cent in Kishanganj to 82–83 per cent in Aizawl and Guntur. CBOs/NGOs and health professionals are reported by a smaller proportion of young women from different districts, but there is growing evidence of identifying them as easy and accessible source of getting male condom.

The cross-sectional data reveals a considerable increase in the proportion of women reporting CBOs/NGOs and health personnel as sources of getting male condoms in the endline survey over the baseline survey.

Table 2.4

Percentage of women knowing at least one source of getting male condom in the five CHARCA districts

Background characteristics	*Kanpur**	*Kishanganj*		*Bellary*		*Guntur*		*Aizawl*	
	EL	*BL*	*EL*	*BL*	*EL*	*BL*	*EL*	*BL*	*EL*
Age (completed years)									
13–16	41.7	43.5	34.5	5.1	61.0	11.3	78.4	25.0	79.8
17–20	71.3	60.8	46.3	11.6	72.0	20.0	84.6	39.4	93.2
21–24	73.4	63.9	49.7	19.4	66.0	30.8	87.2	60.4	96.6
Marital Status									
Married	74.6	63.8	49.2	12.3	65.5	23.2	86.4	67.9	89.1
Unmarried	56.2	49.7	40.1	10.8	67.7	17.4	81.3	36.2	100.0
Women's Education									
Illiterate	52.2	34.6	29.4	2.9	60.7	13.0	73.1	33.3	100.0
<5 years complete	40.0	59.5	41.1	5.8	61.7	—	87.9	29.4	50.0
5–7 years complete	45.8	68.0	50.0	9.2	62.2	16.7	83.9	33.0	84.1
8–9 years complete	53.8	74.5	66.1	12.3	64.6	19.6	80.6	41.1	86.2
10 and above	76.8	89.8	67.2	37.0	80.7	31.2	86.3	48.0	94.9
Husband's Education									
Illiterate	50.0	37.7	41.2	0.0	62.7	14.5	88.0	100.0**	0.0
<5 years complete	66.7	67.7	53.5	21.1	68.4	33.3	90.5	100.0**	0.0
5–7 years complete	56.3	78.8	34.0	8.7	69.8	13.8	84.2	64.7	100.0
8–9 years complete	76.5	72.4	63.3	11.8	68.8	29.4	89.5	66.7	100.0
10 and above	80.5	87.1	70.0	21.2	66.2	36.0	86.5	65.6	100.0
Membership in CBOs/NGOs									
Yes	100.0	66.7	47.8	22.7	85.6	31.9	82.7	50.9	91.9
No	69.8	55.5	66.7	11.2	83.7	18.6	84.9	29.7	84.5
Women's Occupation									
Homemaker	63.2	56.2	44.1	14.6	65.8	24.0	83.7	41.6	90.4
Working as labourer/family farm	45.8	42.1	62.5	4.7	66.1	12.7	85.2	43.9	95.5
Salaried/paid job	71.4	77.8	50.0	23.3	77.4	46.2	100.0	42.1	100.0
Migratory Status of Husband									
Non-migrant	74.2	56.1	42.1	11.8	63.6	20.4	87.1	41.5	100.0
Migrant	68.0	46.2	67.1	0.0	68.9	50.0	83.9	100.0	100.0
Exposure to Mass Media									
Yes	66.1	57.6	48.3	12.8	69	21.7	85.4	41.9	90.9
No	33.3	49.2	35.0	2.0	44.6	14.5	46.2	33.3	100†
Total (N)	62.6 (494)	54.0 (538)	44.9 (465)	11.5 (475)	66.6 (556)	19.7 (471)	84.2 (417)	41.8 (468)	90.9 (439)†

* Information from the baseline survey is not presented due to change in intervention after the survey.

† Less than five cases.

The proportion of young women knowing at least one location to obtain male condom is found to have a positive relationship with age, their education and education of husband.

A relatively higher proportion of married women than their unmarried counterparts reporting knowledge of at least one location of getting male condoms cuts across all the five CHARCA districts. The proportion of such women has increased considerably in all the districts except Kishanganj.

The most striking issue is the significant increase in the proportion of unmarried girls knowing at least one location of getting a male condom in all the districts except Kishanganj. In fact, this commendable achievement confirms the concerted efforts of female peer educators in creating awareness even among young unmarried women.

However, membership in CBOs/NGOs and the main occupation of young women do not reveal a definite pattern in variation in the knowledge of a source of getting male condoms.

As expected, young women in Guntur, Bellary and Aizawl, who are exposed to the media and whose husbands are migrants, are more likely to be aware about the place where condom is available than their counterparts.

Figure 2.1

Percentage of women knowing at least one source of getting condom

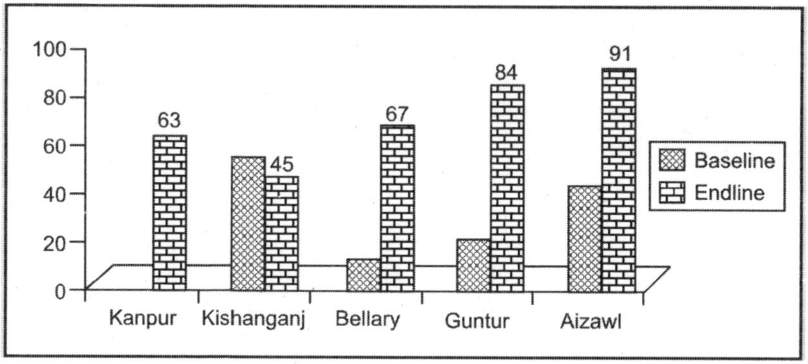

It is clear from the panel data that a majority of the women favoured health personnel as a source of getting male condoms in all the five CHARCA districts, viz., Kanpur, Kishanganj, Bellary, Aizawl and Guntur.

'... condom accessibility is largely seen among the village people which was not the scenario before ... people from villages also buy condom from the local shops. The people also take condom from the village hospital through the ASHA worker ...'

—Woman KI, Kanpur

'... most of the people of the village are using condoms. The awareness about safety of using condom has been increased in this community ... we many time confirm it from local shopkeeper who says about increased condom sell or while discussing about women in meetings where the women report their husbands using condom frequently ...'

—Peer educator FGD, Kishanganj

'... Condom is easily available in the village, however its use is low among the people because of the extra expenditure involved in its purchase. People are poor and many times it is a burden on them to buy condoms each time ...'

—Woman KI, Bellary

'... there are people who save five rupees from their daily basic necessities... people are really poor in this community ... spending five to ten rupees on condom is not affordable to all, when the poverty level is so high they prefer to spend the money on food or medicine rather than buying condom ...'

—Man FGD, Guntur

'... all know about condom in our community. They talk about condom and can say the correct use of condom step-wise what they were told during different meetings and other sessions ... when it comes to uses people think of other alternatives too ... which is cheaper in terms of buying, more convenient in terms of dispose of and storage ...'

—Peer educator, Aizawl

Similar to the survey findings, the qualitative results also revealed that the villagers are using condoms moderately. As observed in the different study sites, condom use is low among the villagers, regardless of its availability or accessibility in shops, etc. Condoms are available in the nearby hospitals and medical shops, but the actual use is quite low among the villagers because villagers think that buying condoms mean extra expenditure, and there is pervasive poverty among the people. Therefore, people show lack of interest in condoms as there is cost involved and they do not want to invest money on such products.

Prevalence of menstrual health problems and treatment-seeking behaviour

A number of recent studies on reproductive health problems in India have highlighted that nearly three-fourths of women in reproductive ages suffer from one or another problems with white discharge and painful menstruation having most commonly. Lack of personal hygiene and unsafe sexual practices are reported to be significantly associated with menstrual problems. In addition, there are many socio-economic and cultural determinants of menstrual problems. Some of the Indian studies have shown a strong association between women's livelihood, work and their reproductive health (Oommen, 2000). In a study of adolescent girls in Rajasthan, it is found that a large proportion of girls were not aware of menstruation when they first experienced it (Khanna and Goyal, 2005). All these studies have further argued that early diagnosis and treatment of menstrual problems is a prerequisite for improving the reproductive health status of women in India. CHARCA interventions have also highlighted the issue of personal hygiene and cleanliness during menstruation among young women. Therefore, information on the same has been collected both in the baseline as well as the endline surveys and may be treated as a proxy variable to assess the demand side of improved services – one among the five pillars of CHARCA. Results are presented in Tables 2.5 and 2.6.

In the baseline as well as endline surveys, young women aged 13–24 were asked whether they have menstrual problems any time during the last 12 months prior to the surveys. It is evident from the data and Figure 2.2 that the prevalence of menstrual problems has significantly declined in Kishanganj and Aizawl but the pattern gets reversed in the case of Bellary and Guntur. However, the reported prevalence is not uniform across different background characteristics. Menstrual problems have a positive relationship with age, occupation, migratory status of husband and exposure to mass media. For instance, women of the older cohort (21–24 years) are more likely to have menstrual problems compared to the younger women aged 13–16. Salaried women in Kanpur, Kishanganj and Bellary were relatively more likely to suffer with menstrual problems during the last 12 months than other women who are either homemakers or working in the family farm. In fact, there is no reason why there should be such a pattern and hence the existing differentials may be due to better reporting of the problem.

Table 2.5

Percentage of women reported to have menstrual problems in the last 12 months prior to the survey in five CHARCA districts by some selected background characteristics

Background characteristics	*Kanpur**	*Kishanganj*		*Bellary*		*Guntur*		*Aizawl*	
	EL	*BL*	*EL*	*BL*	*EL*	*BL*	*EL*	*BL*	*EL*
Age (completed years)									
13–16	18.0	43.4	50.9	28.5	38.0	17.7	25.8	33.3	6.1
17–20	20.5	51.7	48.8	30.2	40.6	25.1	25.6	48.4	2.3
21–24	20.3	52.4	45.0	29.5	49.1	21.8	26.8	36.3	10.1
Marital Status									
Married	17.8	45.9	47.6	27.5	46.7	20.6	25.5	39.6	5.2
Unmarried	20.4	52.8	47.9	30.6	38.2	23.4	26.9	44.0	9.7
Women's Education									
Illiterate	23.9	50.5	42.4	28.3	48.2	26.5	7.7	33.3	0.0
<5 years complete	40.0	46.7	51.1	30.8	38.3	21.7	30.3	62.5	0.0
5–7 years complete	12.0	43.0	53.4	30.3	42.3	24.0	37.1	41.4	4.5
8–9 years complete	18.6	47.3	62.5	35.6	39.0	11.1	16.1	45.7	5.8
10 and above	19.6	61.2	36.1	23.5	38.5	20.4	22.3	33.7	6.3
Husband's Education									
Illiterate	16.7	52.8	37.6	0.00	44.1	24.3	28.0	100.0	0.0
<5 years complete	—	58.1	65.1	42.1	42.1	16.7	19.0	33.3	0.0
5–7 years complete	18.8	48.5	36.0	34.8	60.5	22.4	27.4	47.1	0.0
8–9 years complete	27.5	55.2	70.0	35.3	37.5	11.8	26.3	58.3	22.2
10 and above	12.6	54.2	47.5	32.9	46.2	28.0	24.3	25.0	5.8
Membership in CBOs/NGOs									
Yes	29.4	33.3	34.8	36.4	44.3	25.4	27.3	46.1	5.2
No	24.8	49.1	0.0	29.0	48.2	21.6	26.4	32.7	10.3
Women's Occupation									
Homemaker	19.9	48.0	47.3	29.3	37.5	21.8	24.4	39.2	5.9
Working as labourer/family farm	13.6	73.7	50.0	29.8	48.4	22.4	34.6	56.1	9.1
Salaried/paid job	28.6	44.4	50.0	26.7	54.8	30.8	0.0	31.6	0.0
Migratory Status of Husband									
Non-migrant	19.7	48.4	38.2	29.5	44.2	22.0	25.3	40.4	9.4
Migrant	14.3	57.7	71.4	0.0	50.9	50.0	27.0	33.3	33.3
Exposure to Mass Media									
Yes	20.7	48.2	48.0	29.4	43.4	23.3	26.7	40.2	5.9
No	11.1	51.2	47.0	28.6	32.1	16.0	7.7	66.7	0.0
Total (N)	19.600 (494)	49.0 (538)	47.7 (465)	29.5 (475)	42.3 (556)	22.1 (471)	26.1 (417)	40.4 (468)	5.9 (439)

* Information from the baseline survey is not presented due to change in intervention after the baseline survey.

Figure 2.2

Percentage of women reporting menstrual problem in the last 12 months

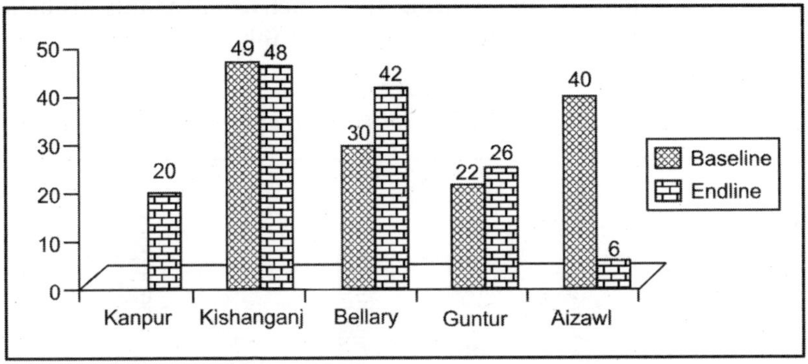

It is found that the reporting about menstrual problems has a positive relationship with the membership of CBOs/NGOs in the entire CHARCA area (Kanpur, Kishanganj, Guntur, Bellary) except Aizawl. Married women from Kishanganj, Bellary and Guntur are more aware about reporting menstrual problems compared to the women from Kanpur and Aizawl. Variation in the reported prevalence of menstrual problems by different socio-economic characteristics brings out two important issues – a higher prevalence of menstrual problems among those belonging to better socio-economic conditions and better reporting by those who are well educated, exposed to media and those

Table 2.6

Percentage of young women (age 13–24 years) seeking treatment for menstrual problems in different health facilities centres in the five CHARCA districts

Different health facility centres	*Kanpur**	*Kishanganj*		*Bellary*		*Guntur*		*Aizawl*	
	EL	*BL*	*EL*	*BL*	*EL*	*BL*	*EL*	*BL*	*EL*
Government hospital	18.7	1.9	15.8	16.1	38.7	8.7	19.3	18.0	50.0
Private hospital	32.7	39.1	47.7	37.8	57.9	38.8	72.5	29.1	31.3
Faith heelers	—	7.1	13.6	1.4†	1.3†	3.4†	0.9†	4.3	—
Home remedy	43.4	38.8	39.3	5.6	13.6	16.9	8.3	43.5	25.0
AYUSH	0.9†	6.6	1.0†	—	1.3†	3.4†	0.9†	0.6†	6.3†
Total Women who reported problems	97	261	222	140	235	103	109	188	26

* Information from the baseline survey is not presented due to change in intervention after the baseline survey.

† Less than five cases.

who have had exposure to different types of programmes and activities. Therefore, the contribution of CHARCA can be marked at least in women experiencing and sharing their menstrual health problems with others, which would have not been possible otherwise.

Figure 2.3

Percentage of women visiting government sector treatment of menstrual problem

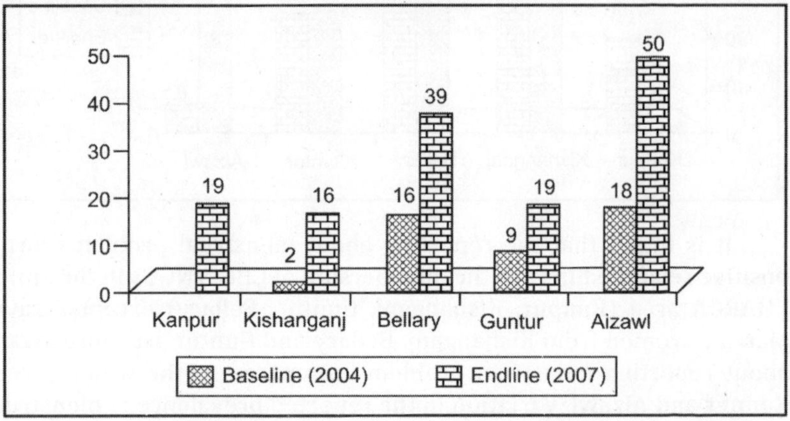

Table 2.6 and Figure 2.3 show the proportion of young women aged 13–24 who had visited health facilities for the treatment of menstruation-related problems. The data reveals that majority of the women in the five CHARCA districts, who reported menstrual problem in the last 12 months, sought treatment mainly from private hospital except Kanpur where a majority of women took home remedy. However, a larger proportion of women in the endline compared with those in the baseline survey reported visiting government hospital/clinic for the treatment of menstrual problems. It is notable here that AYUSH providers are least sought among the five potential places of treatment for menstrual problems in all the five districts. This shows an urgency to address the need to focus on some programmatic interventions which can develop trust in the AYUSH providers as the Government of India has recognized the need to converge reproductive health programme including STI/HIV diagnosis and treatment with the active involvement of AYUSH after training them comprehensively.

The qualitative findings reveal the prevailing culture of silence on matters of women's reproductive and sexual health. The sharing pattern and treatment seeking of reproductive health issues including the menstrual cycle still need attention though the scenario has improved over time.

'... talking about menstruation problems is not that accepted in our village; if an unmarried girl is suffering from any problem related to menstruation, then she first tries to hide it and if problem increases then she discusses it with her friends or mother ...'

—Woman KI, Kishanganj

'... menstrual problem is a widely prevailing phenomenon in women's life everywhere, it is a normal incidence, no need to make the simple problem complicated by taking lots of medicine ... generally girls do not go to see the doctor, rather they go for home treatment only ...'

—Man KI, Guntur

'... in our community girls mostly go for medicines to local shop for their menstrual problems which is quite effective as the salesman is also educated and knows the treatment of many health problems ... hardly someone visits to any doctor for their menstrual problems if the problem is more crucial ...'

—Woman FGD, Aizawl

'... sometimes the girls of our community feel that problems related to irregularity of menstruation are natural and do not need any kind of serious treatment, as a result they even don't discuss about the problems with their mother or someone else in family ...'

—Peer educator FGD, Kanpur

'... most of the women in our village go to quacks for treating the menstrual problems ... they trust the healers as they claim to be specialized in the sexual health problems ... another reason for preferring the quacks is they are easily assessable and not expensive as the allopathic doctors ...'

—Woman KI, Bellary

Regarding treatment-seeking behaviour in case of menstrual problems, it has been reported by earlier studies that women with self-reported symptoms of reproductive morbidity do not seek treatment due to existing taboos and inhibitions regarding sexual and reproductive health. They hesitate to discuss about reproductive problems, especially due to shame and embarrassment (Bang et al., 1989; Oommen, 2000). Therefore, it is a major challenge for the programme to meet the needs of these women by reinforcing demand as well as supply of services. The situation demands more concerted efforts by community-based programmes for rural women where there is a need to create an enabling environment so that a woman feels comfortable to share her problems and may access the treatment as and when required.

Summary of findings and conclusions

Healthcare providers as a source of information on reproductive and sexual health issues to women during the process of their growing up have increased in almost all districts over the baseline survey. Among the other sources of information, a significant decline in the proportion of women who reported friends and peers as the sources of information on reproductive and sexual health in the endline survey reveals an attitudinal change in healthcare providers to interact even with adolescents and youth in the recent years.

- Knowledge of a location of getting male condom by women varies greatly across the five CHARCA districts. There has been a significant increase in the proportion of women in Aizawl and Bellary, who reported medical store, health personnel and NGOs/ CBOs as major locations/places. The percentage of women who reported health personnel as a source of getting male condom increased in all districts except Kanpur. On the other hand, NGOs/CBOs as sources of getting male condom are reported by higher a proportion of women in the endline survey in Bellary, Guntur and Aizawl.
- It is also observed from both the baseline and endline surveys that knowledge of at least one location of getting male condom among the women is higher in three of the five CHARCA districts, namely, Bellary, Guntur and Aizawl. The level of awareness and knowledge about the availability of at least one source of getting male condom has also increased among unmarried women. A relatively larger proportion of women in Guntur, Bellary and Aizawl knew about all the four different locations of getting male condom compared to those in Kanpur and Kishanganj.
- Compared to the CHARCA baseline study, more women exposed to the media reported about menstrual problems in the last 12 months prior to survey in all the CHARCA districts. For treatment of menstrual problems, private hospitals/clinics have been the most preferred sources. However, the proportion of women visiting government hospitals/clinics for the treatment of menstrual problems in the last 12 months has increased in all the CHARCA districts and can be attributed to the efforts made by CHARCA programmes and activities as a part of its mandate to improve reproductive and sexual health services.

3

Awareness and Knowledge about Reproductive and Sexual Health

The need to educate adolescents, particularly the female adolescents, in India, about the different aspects of growing up, has been a huge challenge, more so in the context of existing diverse societal norms across the country. The reproductive health needs of adolescents, which go beyond marriage, healthcare during pregnancy and prevention of diseases, are poorly understood and ill-served, and not addressed by national policies (Jejeebhoy, 1998). Most adolescents are also found to be extremely poorly informed or having patchy knowledge about their own sexuality, physical well-being, bodies, menstruation and physiological changes at puberty, despite the fact that pre-marital sex is not uncommon, even in rural areas, and adolescents lack adequate information to protect from sexually transmitted infections or unwanted pregnancies (Rasheed et al., 1978; Jejeebhoy, 1998; Bhende, 1994; Verma and Lhungdim, 2002; Verma et al., 1997).

Studies have also indicated that during adolescence age, there are many factors that propel adolescents to indulge in risk-taking behaviours, including those towards opposite sex, as they are surrounded by norms and beliefs, outlooks, attitudes and expectations that go beyond their age (Greene et al., 1995; Smith et al., 2002; Goyal, 2005; McManus and Dhar, 2008).

As a part of the CHARCA intervention, comprehensive educational and awareness programmes have been implemented with a mandate to reduce young women's vulnerability to STIs/HIV and to increase the effectiveness of prevention and control of HIV/AIDS in India. These educational programmes focused on enhancing people's knowledge about HIV/AIDS and building behavioural skills to enhance prevention practices. This chapter presents the findings on the current levels of HIV/AIDS knowledge, attitude, and behaviour of the young women and men and changes over the baseline survey. It also discuses about HIV testing among young women and men and their attitude towards people living with HIV/AIDS.

Awareness about HIV/AIDS

All young women and men interviewed were asked if they had ever heard of an illness called HIV/AIDS. Respondents who had heard of AIDS were then asked a series of questions to ascertain the extent of their knowledge. The proportion of women and men who reported that they had heard of HIV/AIDS are shown in Figures 3.1 and 3.2. It is evident from Figure 3.1 that awareness about HIV/AIDS has shown a tremendous improvement in four of the five CHARCA districts over the intervention period. An unexpected pattern in Kanpur has resulted due to a change in the intervention area after the baseline survey and hence it is excluded from the comparative analysis of baseline and endline

Figure 3.1

Percentage of young women who are aware about HIV/AIDS in the five districts of CHARCA project, 2004 and 2007

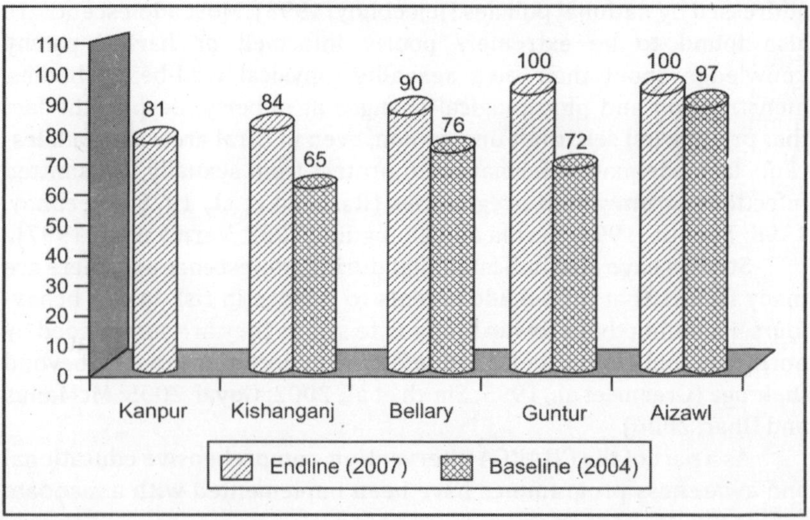

Figure 3.2

Percentage of young men who have heard of HIV/AIDS by district, 2007

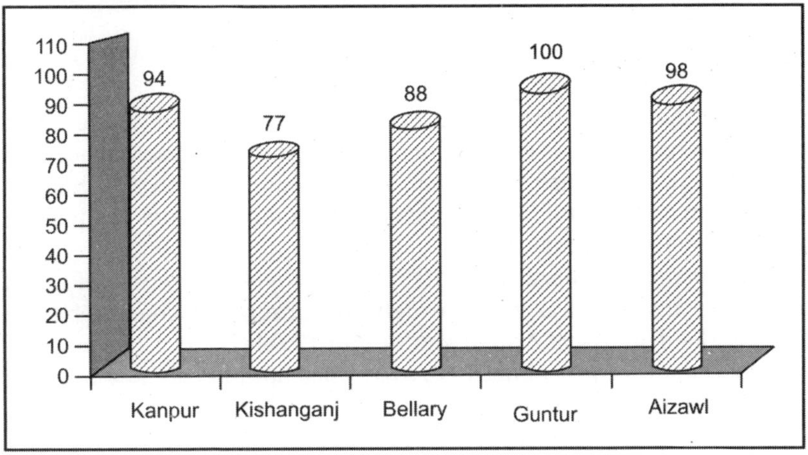

surveys. A large majority of young women and men have reported that they had heard of HIV/AIDS in all the CHARCA districts, including 100 per cent in two districts, namely, Aizawl and Guntur. The overall change in HIV/AIDS awareness among young women during the CHARCA intervention period has been more prominent in Guntur (28%), Kishanganj (19%) and Bellary (14%). Achieving a universal level of awareness about HIV/AIDS even at the time of baseline survey has been the significance in Aizawl district.

The level of awareness about HIV/AIDS among young women is equally high as among young men in all CHARCA districts and even higher than men in Kishanganj. The proportion of women ranges from a minimum in Kanpur (81%) to the maximum in each of Guntur and Aizawl (100%). The level of awareness among women is also high in Bellary (90%) and Kishanganj (84%). The corresponding percentages among young men are 98 per cent in Aizawl, 100 per cent in Guntur, 88 per cent in Bellary, 94 per cent in Kanpur and 77 per cent in Kishanganj. It is worth mentioning that the level of awareness about HIV/AIDS among women as well as men is significantly higher in all the five CHARCA districts than the levels of awareness estimated by NFHS-3. For example, the level of awareness among men and women in Kishanganj, which is having the lowest level of awareness among the five CHARCA districts, is 84 and 77 per cent respectively, which are significantly higher than the NFHS-3 estimates for women (39%) and men (75%) in Bihar. The level of awareness estimated by CHARCA endline is considerably higher than the NFHS-3 estimates except in Aizawl, where CHARCA endline estimates are by and large the same as the NFHS-3 estimates for Mizoram.

A considerable increase in awareness level of HIV/AIDS among young women is also reflected in the case of panel PSUs (8 villages/urban units in each district) between the baseline and endline period. Increasing level of awareness among the respondents included in the panel data also reveals a similar pattern with the highest increase in Kishanganj (32% points), followed by Guntur (23 points) and Bellary (22 points).

Reporting of 'heard about HIV/AIDS' by young women and men across the five districts varies widely by background characteristics, barring the districts of Aizawl and Guntur (Table 3.1a). In Aizawl and Guntur the awareness about HIV/AIDS does not indicate any tangible relationship with the different characteristics as the level is universal. In these two districts every female respondent had heard of HIV/AIDS. However, in the other three districts, namely, Kanpur, Kishanganj and Bellary, background characteristics such as age, marital status, education, residence, occupation and exposure to media have an impact on the awareness level. For instance, the youngest age group (years 13–16) of women reported lower awareness than the other two age groups as in Kanpur (76%), Kishanganj (83%) and Bellary (86%). Young women in their late adolescence (17–20 years) reported higher awareness.

One striking feature that emerged on awareness about HIV/AIDS among young men and women is the influence exerted by social characteristics such as education compared to the demographic or economic characteristics. For instance, illiterates are nearly twice less likely to report awareness than respondents with 10 or more years of education (Table 3.1a). Besides, awareness of HIV/AIDS declines further in Kanpur in the case of young women with illiterate husbands. The proportion aware of HIV/AIDS is 50 per cent in Kanpur, 72 per cent in Kishanganj and 85 per cent in Bellary. In these three districts awareness is lowest among young women with illiterate husbands. The impact of social characteristics, i.e., education, on awareness is found more pronounced in the districts of Kanpur and Bellary for young women and in Kishanganj and Bellary districts for young men (Table 3.1b). In Kanpur, 50 per cent women whose husbands are illiterate were found aware of HIV/AIDS compared to 65 per cent among illiterate young women.

Table 3.1a

Percentage of young women who heard of HIV/AIDS by selected background characteristics

Background characteristics	*Kanpur**	*Kishanganj*		*Bellary*		*Guntur*		*Aizawl*	
	EL	*BL*	*EL*	*BL*	*EL*	*BL*	*EL*	*BL*	*EL*
Age (completed years)									
13–16	75.6	63.2	82.7	74.5	85.7	66.2	100.0	94.8	100.0
17–20	84.1	67.0	86.6	72.4	94.2	69.8	99.4	97.9	100.0
21–24	81.1	63.3	81.7	82.0	88.0	81.2	100.0	97.2	100.0
Marital Status									
Married	75.1	61.6	82.7	76.4	89.3	67.7	100.0	95.2	100.0
Unmarried	83.3	66.8	84.8	76.5	90.3	76.6	99.5	97.1	100.0
Women's Education									
Illiterate	65.2	37.9	64.7	58.4	87.5	56.5	96.2	66.7	100.0
<5 years complete	40.0	66.1	88.9	76.9	85.0	48.0	100.0	81.3	100.0
5–7 years complete	59.3	85.4	93.2	81.7	80.2	63.5	100.0	97.0	100.0
8–9 years complete	80.0	92.7	100.0	86.3	94.0	67.4	100.0	96.3	100.0
10 and above	93.3	100.0	100.0	98.8	99.3	94.9	100.0	98.9	100.0
Husband's Education									
Illiterate	50.0	50.9	71.8	33.3	84.7	55.3	100.0	100.0†	100.0
<5 years complete	100.0	45.2	90.7	84.2	94.7	66.7	100.0	100.0†	100.0
5–7 years complete	62.5	72.7	84.0	71.7	93.0	60.3	100.0	93.8	100.0
8–9 years complete	68.6	75.9	86.7	82.4	93.8	88.2	100.0	95.8	100.0
10 and above	83.9	83.9	92.5	87.1	92.3	86.7	100.0	96.9	100.0
Membership in CBOs/ NGOs									
Yes	100.0	100.0	78.3	90.9	99.6	75.4	99.4	99.6	100.0
No	89.5	64.2	100.0	75.8	99.6	71.2	100.0	93.0	100.0
Women's Occupation									
Homemaker	80.3	65.7	84.1	87.5	90.1	78.8	99.7	96.8	100.0
Working as labourer/family farm	79.2	47.4	68.8	57.3	89.6	60.1	100.0	97.8	100.0
Salaried/paid job	100.0	66.7	100.0	80.0	84.0	76.9	100.0	94.4	100.0
Migratory Status of Husband									
Non-migrant	72.0	64.9	81.5	76.3	89.0	71.7	100.0	96.8	100.0
Migrant	85.7	57.7	85.7	100.0	89.6	100.0	100.0	100.0	100.0
Exposure to Mass Media									
Yes	85.2	73.6	90.2	80.9	91.0	76.3	100	96.8	100.0
No	42.6	33.6	64.1	36.7	73.6	48.7	100	100.0	100.0
Total (N)	80.6 (398)	64.6 (348)	83.7 (389)	76.4 (373)	89.6 (498)	71.8 (339)	99.8 (416)	96.8 (453)	100.0 (439)

* Information from the baseline survey is not presented due to change in intervention after the baseline survey.

† Less than five cases.

Wide differences in awareness were found among respondents in terms of exposure to media and occupation. Among the occupations, both men and women respondents working as labourer in family farm show the lowest awareness level (69% among young women and 74% among young men in Kishanganj, 79% among young women in Kanpur, 86% among young men in Bellary) compared with homemakers or doing salaried/paid jobs (84% in Bellary and universal in the other four districts). Respondents exposed to media also show a higher awareness level: twice higher in Kanpur (85%) and over a quarter per cent higher in Kishanganj (90%).

Table 3.1b

Percentage of men aged 15–29 who have heard of HIV/AIDS

Background characteristics	*Kanpur**	*Kishanganj*		*Bellary*		*Guntur*		*Aizawl*	
	EL	*BL*	*EL*	*BL*	*EL*	*BL*	*EL*	*BL*	*EL*
Age (completed years)									
20 and below	99.3		74.8		82.1		100		97.7
20 plus	99.4		78.0		91.8		100		99.0
Marital Status									
Married	99.2		73.3		91.3		100		100
Unmarried	99.5		79.8		85.5		100		98
Education									
Illiterate	100		55.3		80		100		0.0
<5 years complete	100		73.1		89.3		100		100
5–7 years complete	94.4		83.1		81.8		100		0.0
8–9 years complete	100		87.2		88.6		100		92.3
10 and above	100		93.1		96.5		100		98.8
Membership in CBOs/NGOs									
Yes	100		92.0		100		100		98.2
No	100		92.9		96.7		100		100
Occupation									
Student/not working	100		86.8		92.3		100		98
Working as labourer/ family farm	98.9		74.4		86		100		98
Salaried/paid job	100		77.1		93.5		100		100
Exposure to Mass Media									
Yes	99.4		80.9				100		98.4
No	100†		36.7				100†		0.0
Total (N)	**99.4 (320)**		**76.8 (252)**		**88.0 (279)**		**100 (214)**		**98.4 (181)**

*Information from the baseline survey is not presented due to change in intervention after the baseline survey.

† Less than five cases.

Source of information about HIV/AIDS

CHARCA programmes and activities have been using different forms of media extensively to increase awareness of AIDS and its prevention in the general population. The endline survey asked young women and men who had heard of AIDS to identify the sources from which they learned about AIDS and the results are presented in Tables 3.2a and 3.2b.

Of the many sources of information available to respondents (both men and women) to get information about HIV/AIDS, the media (especially the electronic media) emerged as the main source of information in all the districts, barring Bellary (Karnataka). The proportion of young women that mentioned radio/TV as one of the sources of information ranges from 49 per cent in Bellary, 62 per cent in Kishanganj, 70 per cent in Kanpur, 84 per cent in Guntur to 90 per cent in Aizawl.

Interestingly, to the young women in Bellary, the most commonly mentioned source is the NGOs/CBOs with 63 per cent. Besides Bellary, NGOs/CBOs are also cited by a substantial proportion of young women in Guntur (69%), Aizawl (64%) and Kanpur (30%). Other sources such as posters/hoardings, health professionals and school teachers are not as popular as the media or NGOs/CBOs. However, in Guntur, both health professionals (67%) and posters/hoardings (69%) are also important channels of information on HIV/AIDS to young women.

For young men also, the media is the primary source for HIV/AIDS information. Radio/TV is mentioned by a large majority of young men in Kanpur (98%) and newspapers/magazines by 61 per cent, followed by posters/ hoardings (78%). Radio/TV is mentioned by 64 per cent young men in Kishanganj (25% for newspapers/magazines), and 50 per cent in Bellary (27% for newspapers/magazines). In Bellary, other than the media, the health professionals are also equally prominent as a source of information (51%).

Young men in Aizawl and Guntur get information about HIV/AIDS from more sources besides the media than those in other districts. For instance, in Aizawl, a large majority of young men cited newspapers/magazines (91%), followed by radio/TV (84%), posters/hoardings (77%), NGOs/CBOs (66%), school teachers (65%) and health professionals (48%). Similarly, in Guntur, over four-fifths (83%) mentioned radio/TV and NGOs/CBOs, followed by posters/hoardings (79%), newspapers/magazines (65%) and health professionals (47%), as the main source of information.

Table 3.2a

Percentage of women aged 13–24 who have heard of HIV/AIDS by specific source of information

	Radio/ TV	*Newspaper/ magazines*	*Posture/ hoardings*	*Health professionals*	*School teachers*	*NGOs/ CBOs*
Kanpur*						
EL	**70.2**	**23.9**	**11.3**	**11.7**	**13.2**	**30.2**
Kishanganj						
BL	54.0	14.5	7.1	5.0	8.2	0.7
EL	**62.4**	**13.3**	**1.1**	**28.6**	**4.7**	**1.7**
Bellary						
BL	61.5	25.5	29.8	15.7	24.7	2.9
EL	**48.6**	**23.3**	**23.5**	**31.5**	**25.7**	**62.6**
Guntur						
BL	51.3	34.1	11.6	15.7	27.3	8.5
EL	**83.5**	**31.9**	**68.9**	**66.9**	**25.9**	**69.1**
Aizawl						
BL	51.6	56	21.9	15.7	37.5	31.4
EL	**89.5**	**68.6**	**45.1**	**9.1**	**34.9**	**64.0**

* Information from the baseline survey is not presented due to change in intervention after the baseline survey.

Table 3.2.b

Percentage of men aged 15–29 who have heard of HIV/AIDS by specific source of information (endline)

	Radio/ TV	*Newspaper/ magazines*	*Posture/ hoardings*	*Health professionals*	*School teachers*	*NGOs/ CBOs*
Kanpur						
EL	97.8	60.6	78.1	13.7	11.9	28
Kishanganj						
EL	64	25.3	9.1	8.0	4.0	4.6
Bellary						
EL	49.5	26.5	25.4	50.5	14	43.5
Guntur						
EL	83.2	65	79	47.2	19.6	83.2
Aizawl						
EL	83.7	90.8	77.2	47.8	65.2	66.3

'... We had many serious awareness campaigns efforts by MSAC, PNM (Positive Network Mizoram), etc. Whenever these organizations held awareness campaigns, usually focus is more on the fear factors of HIV/AIDS. They emphasize on the hazardous outcomes of HIV infection in human life course. These programmes are effective, but we should think again, the message should not end there (or be satisfied), but go beyond highlighting the fear factors and give more education that can change the behaviour of people ...'

—Man FGD, Aizawl

'... now a days in any community, be it rural or urban, information on health issues is available from many sources ... how you make it effective is important. Attention should be given to how people would get convinced and accept the message in their behaviour ... rather than repeating the same message under the name of a different organization ...'

—Man KI, Bellary

'... saying one correct thing over and over again is not going to harm anyone, rather it will remind people before behaving ... it's not always possible to touch all at a time ... bringing our new programmatic message is good but we should keep the basic things as they are and we should keep on circulating in the community so that it would fill the gap of reaching as well as it will be echoed in people's mind ...'

—Peer educator, FGD, Kanpur

'... knowledge and information we get on HIV and other health issues is really vital ... the way of conveying the matter is no doubt effective on educationally backward people in our village who don't know how to read and write, making things in play way method and in a simple local language is really helpful ...'

—Men KI, Guntur

'... The people having HIV need lots of support and help, not only form government and other sources but also from their own communities ... so the intervention message should be designed carefully, the message should go beyond the prevention method regarding HIV, it must highlight on sensitizing the people towards the HIV positive people in the community. The programme should aim at creating awareness among the general population without scarring them ...'

—Peer educator, FGD, Kishanganj

Undoubtedly, the media plays a major role in the dissemination of HIV/AIDS information, more so the electronic media. Mere awareness about HIV/AIDS is not sufficient, but certainly an important base to gauge the reach of a programme. Views expressed by concerned local resource persons in FGDs or key informant interviews highlight the need to strategically change the contents of awareness programmes/campaigns. In most districts people feel that the time has come to address issues such as voluntary HIV testing, counselling, reducing stigma and discrimination, care for HIV positive people, etc., rather than on mere information about HIV/AIDS. Such views were echoed during FGDs with young men and young women in Aizawl.

Effectiveness of the efforts made by CHARCA peer educators in enhancing awareness about HIV/AIDS at community level is evident with the fact that a considerable proportion of both women and men in all CHARCA districts, except Kishanganj, reported getting information on HIV/AIDS from CBOs/NGOs and health professionals. The panel data also supports the contribution of health professionals in raising community level awareness about HIV/AIDS. It has been observed during the field work that in a number of cases rural women perceive even the peer educators of CHARCA as health professionals which legitimizes their contribution either as a CHARCA staff or health professionals.

Perception about condom use as protection against HIV/AIDS

Comprehensive awareness about condom use as a means of protection from HIV/AIDS is a prerequisite for reducing women's vulnerability to the epidemic. Every young woman in Aizawl perceives that use of condom can protect a person from acquiring HIV/AIDS, while the proportion is only 28 per cent in Bellary, 42 per cent in Kishanganj, 68 per cent in Kanpur and 97 per cent in Guntur. There has been no significant change in the proportion of young women having this perception, except in Guntur. Guntur district experiences a substantial increase in the proportion (73%).

It is evident from Figures 3.3a and 3.3b that a fairly large proportion of young women and young men perceive that using condom consistently during each sexual intercourse can prevent HIV/AIDS. Over three-fifths of young women in each district perceive that consistent condom use in every sexual intercourse can prevent HIV/AIDS. The proportion of such women are 75 per cent in Kishanganj, 90 per cent in Kanpur, 95 per cent in Bellary, 97 per cent in Guntur and 100 per cent in Aizawl.

Figure 3.3a

Percentage of young women who perceive use of condom as protection against HIV/AIDS, 2004–2007

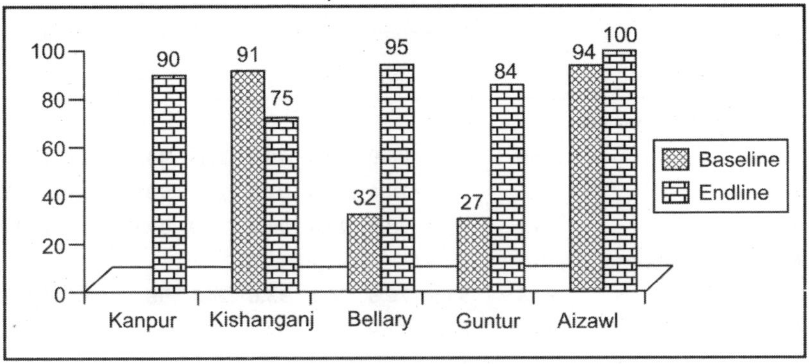

Figure 3.3b

Percentage of young men who perceive use of condom as protection against HIV/AIDS, 2004–2007

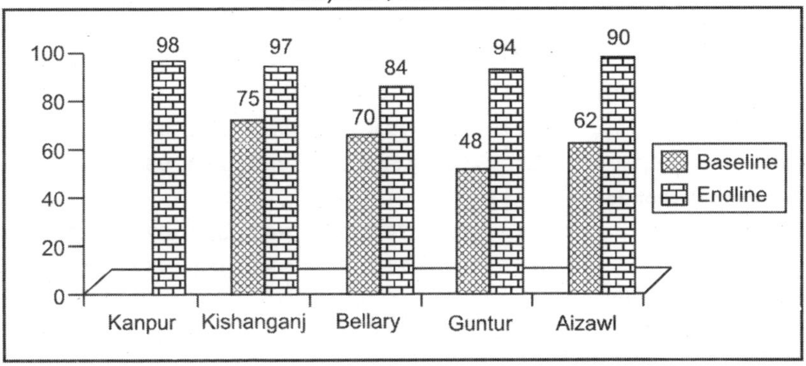

Compared to the baseline results, the increase in the proportion of young women perceiving consistent condom use as protection against HIV/AIDS has been substantially high in Bellary and Guntur. However, these proportions are significantly higher than those estimated in NFHS-3 for the respective states. For example, a young woman in Kishanganj (having the lowest proportion of young women perceiving consistent condom use as protection against HIV/AIDS among five CHARCA districts) is three times more likely than a woman aged 15–24 in Bihar as estimated by NFHS-3. The same is considerably higher even in other CHARCA districts. Thus, a comparison of the state level estimates of youth's perception about consistent condom use as

Table 3.3a

Percentage of women knowing that consistent use of condom during each sexual intercourse can protect from HIV infections

Background characteristics	*Kanpur**	*Kishanganj*		*Bellary*		*Guntur*		*Aizawl*	
	EL	*BL*	*EL*	*BL*	*EL*	*BL*	*EL*	*BL*	*EL*
Age (completed years)									
13–16	83.9	87.8	76.9	20.6	90.4	17.3	94.8	96.1	100.0
17–20	91.5	92.4	70.4	33.6	91.8	28.3	98.1	92.3	100.0
21–24	93.1	91.6	78.8	43.0	94.0	33.9	97.0	93.5	100.0
Marital Status									
Married	91.3	93.6	76.6	34.1	93.6	24.4	98.0	97.4	100.0
Unmarried	88.9	88.5	73.9	29.0	90.4	29.4	95.6	93.1	100.0
Women's Education									
Illiterate	66.7	83.8	70.9	18.8	93.2	08.7	100.0	100.0†	100.0
<5 years complete	75.0	91.3	75.0	30.8	82.4	04.0	97.0	83.3	
5–7 years complete	80.0	95.5	69.5	27.0	95.5	19.0	98.4	93.8	100.0
8–9 years complete	90.5	84.3	78.6	33.3	92.2	26.1	90.3	95.5	100.0
10 and above	94.7	98.0	88.5	53.8	92.0	49.0	97.8	93.0	100.0
Membership in CBOs/NGOs									
Yes	94.1	83.3	77.8	52.6	95.7	23.2	97.8	93.3	100.0
No	92.2	90.7	100.0	30.9	96.5	27.3	96.2	94.6	100.0
Women's Occupation									
Homemaker	90.3	90.6	74.5	35.2	90.7	31.8	97.6	93.9	100.0
Working as labourer/family farm	78.9	88.9	72.7	21.4	93.6	18.5	93.8	97.5	100.0
Salaried/paid job	85.7	100.0	90.0	41.7	96.2	23.1†	100.0	83.3	100.0
Migratory Status of Husband									
Non-migrant	90.5	91.0	72.4	32.0	93.4	26.6	97.2	93.8	100.0
Migrant	91.7	80.0	86.7	33.3	93.7	50.0†	100.0	100.0†	100.0
Exposure to Mass Media									
Yes	82.6	90.3	77.4	32.5	92.3	30.8	97.3	93.8	100.0
No	90.1	92.7	66.7	22.2†	87.8	05.3†	84.6	100.0	100.0
Total (N)	**89.7 (398)**	**90.5 (349)**	**75.3 (389)**	**32.0 (372)**	**92.0 (498)**	**26.7 (472)**	**96.9 (416)**	**93.8 (453)**	**100.0 (439)**

* Information from the baseline survey is not presented due to change in intervention after the baseline survey.

† Less than five cases.

protection against HIV/AIDS and the estimates of CHARCA endline survey point to a clear impact of CHARCA programmes and activities in enhancing comprehensive awareness among young women as well as young men.

It is evident from Table 3.3a that a considerable proportion of young women aged 13–16, illiterate, unmarried, working as labourers and not exposed to media are less likely to be aware that consistent use

Table 3.3b

Percentage of men knowing that consistent use of condom during each sexual intercourse can protect from HIV infections (endline)

Background characteristics	*Kanpur*	*Kishanganj*	*Bellary*	*Guntur*	*Aizawl*
Age (completed years)					
20 and below	97.4	97.8	81.2	95.7	98.9
20+	98.8	96.9	86.0	93.8	99.0
Marital Status					
Married	98.4	95.5	83.0	95.4	100.0
Unmarried	97.9	98.6	85.7	92.7	98.7
Education					
Illiterate	100.0*	98.3	75.0	0.0	0.0
<5 years complete	90.5	84.2	88.0	85.7	100.0*
5–7 years complete	100.0	94.4	73.3	95.7	0.0
8–9 years complete	98.0	100.0	80.6	100.0	100.0
10 and above	98.8	100.0	94.5	93.8	98.8
Membership in CBOs/NGOs					
Yes	100.0	100.0	87.5	90.5	98.8
No	98.1	100.0	87.9	95.5	100.0
Occupation					
Students/not working	97.0	98.3	98.1	93.9	99.0
Working as labourer/family farm	98.3	97.5	82.6	95.0	98.0
Salaried/paid job	100.0	95.9	72.4	92.3	100.0
Exposure to Mass Media					
Yes	98.1	97.1	84.1	94.3	98.9
No	100.0	100.0	85.7	100.0*	0.0
Total	98.1	97.2	84.2	94.4	98.9
Total Respondents	**320**	**252**	**279**	**214**	**184**

* Less than five cases.

of condom during each sexual intercourse can protect a person against HIV. However, the gap in such awareness among young women is found to be wider by exposure to media and education, especially in Kanpur and Kishanganj. For instance, in Kanpur, 67 per cent illiterate women compared to 95 per cent with 10 or more years, education perceived that consistent use of condom during each sexual intercourse can protect a person against HIV. In Kishanganj, the gap is 19 percentage points between the two groups. Similarly, in these two districts, and also in Guntur, women with exposure to media reported a higher level of awareness (9–12%).

The increase in perception about correct condom use among young women is also high in the panel PSUs compared to baseline levels. For instance, Guntur and Bellary reported a substantial increase of over 44 percentage points, while in Aizawl the level remains the same (100%). In other two districts (Kishanganj and Kanpur) the levels show a decrease in the proportion of young women who believe condom use can prevent HIV/AIDS.

Table 3.3b shows that most of the young men aged 15–29 are aware that the use of condom can protect a person from acquiring STIs and HIV/AIDS. Nine in ten young men in Aizawl, Kanpur and Guntur perceive that condom can protect a person from both STI and HIV. The proportion is much lower in Kishanganj where 63 per cent perceive condoms as protective measure against STIs and 75 per cent against HIV/AIDS. Compared to the baseline results, each district records a substantial increase in the proportion of young men who are aware of condom use as protection against STIs or HIV/AIDS. Among the districts, Guntur shows the highest increase in the proportion of such young men, i.e., 52 per cent for STIs and 49 per cent for HIV/AIDS.

The importance of condom, despite its low use in all the districts, is also expressed strongly by many young men. For example, interactions with young men through focus group discussions or as key informants clearly bring out the benefits condom has as a protective measure against STIs/HIV. In one such interaction with young men in Aizawl, they vehemently stressed the need to carry condom and use it in each sexual intercourse as it is now easily available in shops and also freely distributed by NGOs and government agencies.

Preventive measures for HIV/AIDS and STIs

Young women were also asked about their perceptions of other measures to prevent STIs and HIV/AIDS. The survey vividly brings out the depth and expansion in awareness and knowledge young women

'... there are many women easily available on the streets for men. To go to these women is always risky. So, unless we know women very well, the best thing for men is to avoid sex with such women, which is the safest. But once some one wants to have sex with them, then condom is a must ...'

—Man FGD, Aizawl

'... most of the men in our village know that condom is safe against HIV... I have heard other women saying that the husbands talking about the condom's benefits to them ... they share the knowledge and information they get from their husband and other women at gossip during water collection or any other leisure occasion ...'

—Woman FGD, Guntur

'... though it is a bit embarrassing, we talk about safety measures regarding sexual life, condom use, treatment of sexual health problems while we do some chit chat in groups, particularly to those people whom we know to go for some relationships other than their wives ... who knows, our talk may save some one's life ...'

—Man KI, Kanpur

'... I feel condom is must when going for sex with everyone other than your wife or girl friend. Earlier I thought the condom is only to be used if you are going to brothels but we cant make out from the outer appearance of a person about her status. So avoiding condom may be fatal some time ...'

—Man KI, Bellary

'... some say condom hampers the fun in sex ... but what is important, life or fun ... it's we to decide ... I will use condom if I go for sex out side of marriage even if it really reduces the pleasure.'

—Man KI, Kishanganj

have about STIs/HIV over the years in the five survey districts. The impact of intervention is clearly visible in Kishanganj, Bellary and Guntur. In these three districts, there has been a substantial increase in the proportion of young men knowing about preventive measures compared to the baseline results of 2004 (Table 3.4a). Overall, only Aizawl district has achieved universal level in awareness and knowledge about HIV/STI measures, but Guntur district tops in the most substantial increase.

It is evident from Tables 3.4a and 3.4b that a majority of young women and men know that 'checking blood prior to transfusion' is a preventive measure for HIV/AIDS. The proportion of such young women ranges from 76 per cent in Kanpur to 100 per cent in Aizawl. In other districts, the proportion is as high as 98 per cent in Guntur, 88 per cent in Bellary and 81 per cent in Kishanganj. The corresponding proportion of young men is 95 per cent in Kanpur, 99 per cent in Aizawl, 95 per cent in Bellary, 96 per cent in Guntur and 96 per cent in Kishanganj. In the case of changes in the proportion of women having such knowledge (men were not asked this question in the baseline survey), Guntur shows the highest increase of 50 per cent over the CHARCA intervention period. Similarly, in the case of other measures such as 'sterilizing needles and syringes for injections', 'avoiding sex with CSW' and 'sex with only one partner', all the districts recorded a substantial increase in the proportion of young women perceiving them as preventive measures against HIV. Again, Aizawl stands out for reporting universal level, followed by Guntur for near universal level (97–99%). In the case of 'sex with only one partner', the proportion ranges from 66 per cent in Bellary to 100 per cent in Aizawl. Mention may be made of Kishanganj district which recorded the highest increase among the districts with 52 per cent over the baseline survey.

Table 3.4a

Percentage of women by their perception about some measures for HIV/AIDS prevention in the five CHARCA districts

Background characteristics	*Kanpur**	*Kishanganj*		*Bellary*		*Guntur*		*Aizawl*	
	EL N=398	*BL N=538*	*EL N=389*	*BL N=487*	*EL N=556*	*BL N=472*	*EL N=416*	*BL N=453*	*EL N=439*
Preventive measures									
Checking blood prior to transfusion	**75.7**	60.7	**80.7**	70.1	**87.6**	49.4	**97.8**	93.6	**100.0**
Sterilizing needles and syringes for injection	**76.0**	59.2	**72.0**	69.1	**87.6**	47.5	**98.6**	93.4	**100.0**
Avoid sex with CSW	**72.7**	44.7	**84.3**	68.2	**86.3**	53.2	**96.9**	91.3	**100.0**
Sex with only one partner	**70.4**	40.8	**84.8**	69.3	**66.4**	51.8	**99.0**	84.7	**99.8**

* Information from the baseline survey is not presented due to change in intervention after the baseline survey.

For men, though there is no comparative figures from the baseline, the endline estimates for these proportions reveal extremely higher proportions of men aware of these preventive measures (Table 3.4b).

Table 3.4b

Percentage of men by their perception about some measures for HIV/AIDS prevention in the five CHARCA district (endline)

Preventive measures	*Kanpur*	*Kishanganj*	*Bellary*	*Guntur*	*Aizawl*
Checking blood prior to transfusion	95.3	96.4	95.3	95.8	98.9
Sterilizing needles and syringes for injection	97.5	93.7	84.9	96.7	100.0
Avoid sex with CSW	96.9	93.3	97.1	94.9	85.6
Sex with only one partner	93.4	93.3	93.9	93.0	98.9
Total Men	**320**	**252**	**279**	**214**	**181**

Table 3.5a

Percentage of women by perceptions about STI prevention in the five CHARCA districts

Preventive measures	*Kanpur*	*Kishanganj*		*Bellary*		*Guntur*		*Aizawl*	
	EL	*BL*	*EL*	*BL*	*EL*	*BL*	*EL*	*BL*	*EL*
Using condom consistently in each sexual intercourse	**63.0**	73.8	**68.5**	5.2	**52.2**	9.7	**91.4**	67.7	**90.4**
Sex with only one partner	**57.1**	68.5	**74.4**	9.2	**47.8**	16.3	**91.8**	65.0	**90.4**
Avoid sex with CSW	**62.6**	57.1	**82.7**	9.2	**52.0**	16.7	**91.1**	68.6	**86.1**
Total Women heard about RTIs/STIs	**70.4 (494)**	83.9 (539)	**83.2 (465)**	12.1 (488)	**58 (556)**	19.5 (472)	**93.3 (417)**	73.5 (468)	**90.4 (439)**

Table 3.5a and 3.5b present the perceptions that young women and young men have with regard to prevention measures of STIs. It is evident from these tables that in the cases of both women and men there has been a considerable increase in the proportion of youths who perceive that 'using condom consistently in each sexual intercourse' can protect a person from STIs. There is also an increase in the proportion of respondents even in case of other preventive measures of STIs, but the levels are relatively lower than that of HIV. Guntur and

Bellary show the maximum overall increase in the proportion of female as well as male respondents who are aware of protective measures of STIs over the CHARCA intervention periods. For instance, the increase in the proportion of young women has been 90 per cent in Bellary and 89 per cent in Guntur, who perceive using condom consistently in each sexual intercourse as preventive measure against STIs.

Table 3.5b

Men's perception about condoms as means of protection against STIs/HIV in the five CHARCA districts

Perceptions from infections	*Kanpur**	*Kishanganj*		*Bellary*		*Guntur*		*Aizawl*	
	EL	*BL*	*EL*	*BL*	*EL*	*BL*	*EL*	*BL*	*EL*
Use of condom can protect a person from acquiring STI	**99.0**	50.9	**63.1**	81.6	**94.5**	47.0	**96.5**	71.8	**91.8**
Use of condom can protect a person from acquiring HIV	**98.1**	74.6	**75**	69.9	**84.2**	48.1	**94.4**	61.8	**98.9**
Avoiding pregnancy when one has been tested for HIV can protect one person from getting STI	**82.6**	†	**53**	†	**85.5**	†	**88.3**	†	**87.5**
Avoiding pregnancy when one has been tested for HIV can protect one person from getting HIV	**79.4**	†	**64.6**	†	**81.0**	†	**94.4**	†	**92.9**
Total Men	**322**	291	**328**	256	**317**	264	**214**	220	**184**

* Information from the baseline survey is not presented due to change in intervention after the baseline survey.
† Not asked in the baseline study.

In the case of panel PSUs, the baseline and endline results of young women's perceptions about selected preventive measures of HIV/AIDS and RTIs/STIs show a mixed level. In the case of HIV/AIDS measures, compared to the baseline survey more young women in Aizawl, Guntur and Bellary perceived that checking blood prior to transfusion and sterilizing needles and syringes for injection can prevent HIV/AIDS. But, in the case of perception about avoiding unprotected sex with CSWs as preventing HIV/AIDS, all the districts show an increase in perception, barring Aizawl, which shows a marginal decrease (3%). Similarly, in the case of RTIs/STIs also, more young women in Guntur, Bellary and Kishanganj than in Kanpur or Aizawl show higher increase in perceptions about RTI/STI preventive measures such as sex with one partner, using condom correctly and avoiding sex with CSWs.

However, despite the overall improvement in awareness about the preventive measures of STIs/HIV, there is a sizeable proportion of young women in each group who are still ignorant of some of the important protective measures. Hence, similar programmes and activities are extremely important for enhancing the overall awareness of young women in rural areas which can negatively affect their vulnerability to STIs/HIV.

Misconceptions about acquiring HIV/AIDS

Tables 3.6a and 3.6c present the levels of misconceptions young women and young men have regarding modes of HIV/AIDS transmissions in each of the five districts. The modes pertain to acquiring HIV/AIDS from an HIV positive person by shaking hands, hugging, kissing, through sex, sharing clothes/utensils/shaving blades, bites from bugs/fleas/mosquitoes and stepping on urine/stool of HIV positive persons. The survey indicates a drastic decrease in misconceptions about the different modes, as more young women have acquired correct knowledge of HIV/AIDS transmission during the CHARCA intervention period (Figure 3.4). Of course, one cannot have a

Figure 3.4

Proportion of young women having at least one misconception about mode of HIV/AIDS transmission, 2004 and 2007

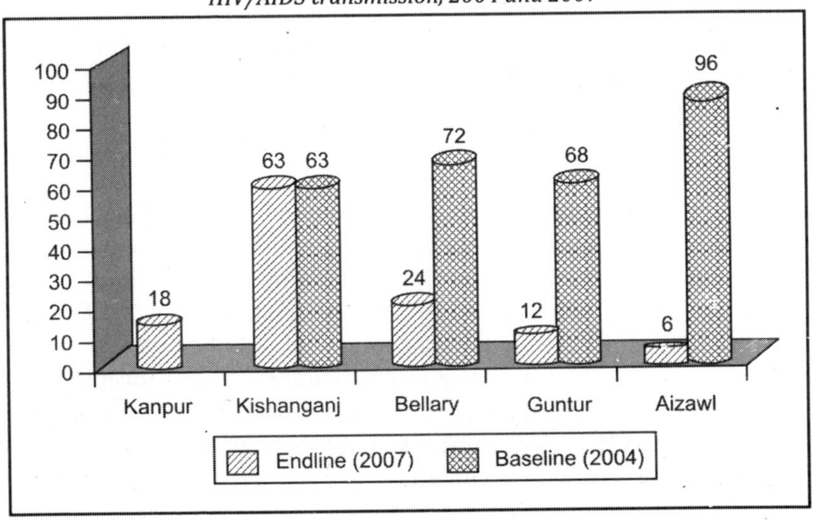

comparative picture for young women in Kanpur and men from either of the five districts. But the pattern in misconceptions clearly shows that a relatively larger proportion of young men have at least one misconception. This means that the CHARCA programmes and activities have primarily benefited young women, at least in the case of imparting correct knowledge and eliminating misconceptions. The percentage change in the proportion of young women with no misconceptions in the last three years (baseline survey) is 96 per cent in Aizawl, 91 per cent in Kanpur, 64 per cent in Guntur and 58 per cent in Bellary. Kishanganj district has shown no change since 2004 (37%).

A drastic decrease indicated in the proportion of young women with at least one misconception about HIV/AIDS in all the districts except Kishanganj reinforces the effectiveness of the awareness programmes organized under CHARCA intervention either through one to one or one to group counselling of peer educators. For instance, the proportion of women with at least one misconception in the endline survey has been reduced to 6 per cent from 96 per cent in Aizawl, 12 per cent from 68 per cent in Guntur and 24 per cent from 72 per cent in Bellary though there in no achievement in Kishanganj where 63 per cent of young women included in the endline survey still carry at least one misconception (the same level as estimated in the baseline survey).

The most common misconception young women have about modes of acquiring HIV/AIDS pertains to 'bites by mosquitoes'. The proportion is 3 per cent in Aizawl, 6 per cent in Guntur (also for stepping on urine/stool), 9 per cent in Kanpur, 18 per cent in Bellary and 35 per cent in Kishanganj. Misconception about kissing is also high in Kishanganj (27%) and Bellary (14%).

As shown in Table 3.6b, misconception is more prominent among young women with certain background characteristics such as age, residence, occupation, etc. Young women who are more likely to have at least one misconception about acquiring HIV/AIDS than others are in the age group 21–24, illiterates, non-members of CBOs/NGOs, and those having no exposure to media. Other characteristics show no discernible difference in misconception. In Kanpur, women in late adolescence (17–20 years) reported a higher level misconception. The differential in misconceptions by residence is also not considerable despite the fact that most rural residents show higher levels. A similar pattern is also true with occupation.

Table 3.6a

Percentage of women having misconceptions about acquiring HIV/AIDS from different modes in the five CHARCA districts, 2004 and 2007

Mode of acquiring HIV/AIDS	*Kanpur**	*Kishanganj*		*Bellary*		*Guntur*		*Aizawl*	
	Extent of misconceptions								
	EL	*BL*	*EL*	*BL*	*EL*	*BL*	*EL*	*BL*	*EL*
Shaking hand	**1.2**	2.4	**1.8**	22.1	**1.2**	7.8	**1.7**	5.9	—
Hugging	**1.3**	2.2	**2.1**	29.7	**1.4**	11.0	**1.0**	7.0	—
Kissing	**2.3**	36.9	**27.0**	36.9	**14.1**	14.8	**1.2**	48.2	**2.5**
Sharing clothes	**3.6**	7.2	**8.7**	28.7	**2.6**	10.8	**4.6**	16.6	**0.2**
Sharing eating utensils	**3.4**	7.1	**9.0**	39.3	**5.6**	12.1	**2.9**	12.5	—
Stepping on urine/ stool	**3.0**	11.0	**17.0**	30.1	**11.2**	17.6	**5.8**	23.1	—
Bites by mosquito/flea/ bedbug	**9.3**	22.4	**35.0**	48.0	**17.5**	23.9	**5.5**	48.0	**3.2**
No misconceptions	**81.7**	37.3	**36.8**	28.3	**67.3**	32.0	**88**	3.8	**94.3**
At least one misconception	**18.3**	62.7	**63.0**	71.7	**23.7**	68.0	**11.8**	96.2	**5.7**

* Information from the baseline survey is not presented due to change in intervention after the baseline survey.

Table 3.6b

Percentage of women having at least one misconception of HIV/AIDS

Background characteristics	*Kanpur**	*Kishanganj*		*Bellary*		*Guntur*		*Aizawl*	
	EL	*BL*	*EL*	*BL*	*EL*	*BL*	*EL*	*BL*	*EL*
Age (completed years)									
13–16	**13.6**	60.6	**53.8**	68.6	**37.2**	60.9	**13.4**	94.1	**10.5**
17–20	**22.0**	65.3	**62.0**	67.3	**29.2**	66.8	**8.3**	97.3	**6.2**
21–24	**18.1**	62.1	**69.2**	78.4	**32.7**	77.4	**14.0**	96.5	**1.4**
Marital Status									
Married	**19.7**	59.8	**69.8**	72.5	**30.9**	64.6	**10.6**	92.0	**6.5**
Unmarried	**17.8**	64.8	**55.4**	70.6	**34.2**	72.0	**13.2**	96.9	**1.4**
Women's Education									
Illiterate	**13.3**	37.0	**66.4**	54.9	**39.5**	50.4	**15.4**	66.7	**0.0**
<5 years complete	**25.0**	62.8	**62.5**	75.0	**35.3**	48.0	**12.1**	70.6	**0.0**
5–7 years complete	**28.6**	83.5	**67.1**	73.4	**28.1**	60.3	**10.5**	97.0	**13.6**
8–9 years complete	**19.0**	92.7	**57.1**	78.1	**29.9**	63.0	**14.5**	95.7	**5.1**
10 and above	**16.7**	95.9	**57.4**	97.5	**29.1**	92.4	**10.8**	98.9	**4.7**

Cont'd...

...Cont'd

Husband's Education									
Illiterate	**0.0**	49.1	**65.6**	33.3†	**31.0**	52.6	**20.0**	100.0†	**0.0**
<5 years complete	**0.0**	41.9	**79.5**	84.2	**33.3**	58.3	**9.5**	100.0†	**0.0**
5–7 years complete	**10.0**	72.7	**64.3**	65.2	**45.0**	53.4	**8.4**	88.2	**0.0**
8–9 years complete	**31.4**	75.9	**88.5**	79.4	**6.7**	88.2	**10.5**	95.8	**0.0**
10 and above	**17.8**	83.9	**59.5**	83.5	**26.7**	85.3	**10.8**	93.8	**1.9**
Membership in CBOs/NGOs									
Yes	**11.8**	100.0	**66.7**	86.4	**21.3**	72.5	**10.2**	99.3	**3.9**
No	**16.3**	62.3	**66.7**	71.0	**25.4**	67.2	**12.3**	92.1	**17.2**
Women's occupation									
Homemaker	**18.8**	63.7	**62.0**	82.9	**33.0**	75.3	**10.2**	96.1	**6.1**
Working as labourer/family farm	**15.8**	47.4	**100**	52.0	**32.6**	55.5	**17.3**	97.6	**0.0**
Salaried/paid job	**0.0**	66.7	**40.0**	76.7	**30.8**	76.9	**25.0**	94.7	**0.0**
Migratory Status of Husband									
Non-migrant	**20.0**	63.0	**67.6**	71.5	**34.3**	67.9	**12.4**	96.2	**0.0**
Migrant	**12.5**	57.7	**75.0**	100.0†	**26.3**	100.0†	**5.4**	100.0	**0.0**
Exposure to Mass Media									
Yes	**18.1**	71.7	**72.0**	76.3	**33.0**	73.5	**11.6**	96.2	**5.7**
No	**21.7**	32.0	**60.8**	30.6	**29.3**	39.5	**15.4**	100.0	**0.0**
Total (N)	**18.3 (398)**	62.7 (539)	**63.0 (389)**	71.7 (488)	**29.3 (556)**	68.0 (472)	**11.8 (417)**	96.2 (468)	**5.7 (439)**

* Information from the baseline survey is not presented due to change in intervention after the baseline survey.
† Less than five cases.

Table 3.6c

Percentage of men having misconceptions about acquiring HIV/AIDS from different modes in the five CHARCA districts, 2004 and 2007

Mode of acquiring HIV/AIDS	*Kanpur*	*Kishanganj*	*Bellary*	*Guntur*	*Aizawl*
Shaking hand	2.5	4.7	1.4	0.0	0.5
Hugging	2.8	4.7	1.1	0.5	0.5
Kissing	8.4	17.8	12.9	6.5	2.2
Sharing clothes	6.9	21.7	2.5	2.8	0.0
Sharing eating utensils	11.6	19.0	9.0	1.4	0.0
Stepping on urine/ stool	10.3	12.6	14.0	3.3	1.1
Bites by mosquito/flea/ bedbug	40.3	35.6	31.9	16.8	4.9
No misconceptions	24.8	32.3	45.4	50.9	88.0
At least one misconception	62.7	39.9	42.3	49.1	11.4

The salaried persons are more likely to have misconceptions than others in Guntur, homemakers in Kanpur and Bellary and among labourers in Kishanganj. Exposure to media shows considerable variation in misconceptions. Those not exposed to media have a higher level of at least one misconception about HIV/AIDS. The role played by the media in creating awareness is not confined to HIV alone, but is more prominent as a source in Kishanganj.

When compared to the baseline results, the present levels show a significant improvement in reduction of misconceptions about HIV/AIDS in all the districts. Even among young women with no exposure to media the proportion with at least one misconception has reduced largely, except in Kishanganj. Improvement in the level of misconception is also reflected in the case of panel PSUs over the baseline results: young women in Kishanganj (an increase of 32% points), Aizawl (20% points) and Bellary (16% points). Guntur shows no change over the period in the proportion with at least one misconception (56%).

HIV testing among youth

Over the years, India has continuously been establishing an increasing number of voluntary counselling and testing centres in order to strengthen the reach and coverage of the testing. In fact, one of the major challenges of the HIV prevention programme in India is the ignorance and denial of HIV risk, especially among youth. More than two-fifths of youth in India believe that they are not vulnerable to HIV although there is growing evidence of increased risky sexual behaviour among youth (NACO, 2004). In addition, young people, particularly unmarried youth, often face barriers in accessing reproductive health services, particularly services relating to sexual health. As a result, youth are less likely to have their HIV status tested despite the increasing number of VCT centres across the country. To obtain information on the prevalence of HIV testing, all respondents in CHARCA endline survey were asked whether they had ever been tested for HIV/AIDS. While asking this question, it was clearly specified that the interviewer did not have any intention to know the test results. Respondents who said that they had ever been tested were further asked whether they were tested in the last 12 months. All those who reported that they were never tested for HIV/AIDS were asked whether they knew of a place where one can get tested. The results of the responses to these questions on HIV testing are presented in Tables 3.7 and 3.8 respectively.

Table 3.7

Percentage of women aged 13–24 who reported ever tested for HIV and were tested in the last 12 months, and among those who never tested for HIV, those knowing at least one place for HIV testing by selected background characteristics in CHARCA districts

Background characteristics	*Kanpur*			*Kishanganj*			*Bellary*			*Guntur*			*Aizawl*		
	1	*2*	*3*	*1*	*2*	*3*	*1*	*2*	*3*	*1*	*2*	*3*	*1*	*2*	*3*
Age (completed years)															
13–16	20.3	100.0	59.6	5.5	80.0	44.2	11.0	47.1	62.6	3.1	66.7	89.4	—	—	94.7
17–20	18.3	100.0	69.4	6.3	77.8	48.5	34.4	56.7	63.3	34.8	66.7	96.0	12.4	72.7	96.1
21–24	19.8	25.0	63.4	9.6	93.3	42.4	54.4	55.0	61.2	55.5	41.8	93.2	30.4	42.2	96.1
Marital Status															
Married	19.0	25.0	60.2	12.7	84.6	40.7	53.6	49.6	58.3	60.0	49.6	90.4	44.4	46.9	97.5
Unmarried	19.6	100.0	67.3	1.6	100.0	49.4	13.8	69.4	64.7	3.9	85.7	94.3	9.5	57.1	95.5
Women's Education															
Illiterate	10.0	—	48.1	11.8	76.9	21.9	36.7	50.0	55.9	52.0	61.5	75.0	—	—	100.0
<5 years complete	—	—	25.0	6.3	100.0	38.7	35.3	55.6	54.5	54.5	44.4	90.0	—	—	100.0
5–7 years complete	28.6	100.0	44.0	7.3	83.3	44.7	29.2	46.2	68.3	41.9	55.8	94.4	6.8	33.3	92.7
8–9 years complete	20.7	—	58.7	7.1	100.0	66.0	22.1	58.8	60.0	16.1	50.0	90.4	11.6	43.8	93.4
10 and above	19.1	66.7	75.7	1.6	100.0	73.3	36.6	63.3	70.6	26.6	48.6	96.1	18.9	56.3	97.6
Husband's Education															
Illiterate	16.7	—	80.0	9.8	100.0	29.6	48.0	45.8	59.6	56.0	42.9	81.8	—	—	—
<5 years complete	—	—	33.3	25.6	80.0	41.4	61.1	72.7	71.4	61.9	46.2	87.5	—	—	—
5–7 years complete	40.0	—	33.3	7.1	66.7	23.7	52.5	43.0	58.0	63.2	48.3	94.3	100.0	—	—

Cont'd...

...Cont'd

8–9 years complete	11.4	—	58.1	7.7	100.0	58.3	60.0	44.4	66.7	68.4	46.2	100.0	33.3	66.7	100.0
10 and above	20.5	33.3	63.8	13.5	80.0	65.6	60.0	52.8	50.0	55.4	56.1	87.9	46.2	45.8	96.4
Place of Residence															
Urban	—	—	—	9.5	90.0	44.7	33.3	57.1	60.7	33.6	48.6	93.2	16.7	60.5	95.8
Rural	19.3	57.1	65.0	6.7	84.2	45.2	33.0	54.7	62.7	36.3	52.3	92.8	13.2	37.5	95.6
Membership in CBOs/NGOs															
Yes	17.6	—	64.3	11.1	100.0	62.5	45.7	53.5	74.5	46.1	46.3	90.6	16.0	52.5	96.3
No	18.4	60.0	73.9	—	—	66.7	31.0	48.1	69.5	28.3	56.7	93.4	10.3	50.0	92.3
Women's Occupation															
Homemaker	19.1	50.0	66.1	6.9	88.0	44.0	31.7	61.1	63.4	34.4	57.0	92.6	13.5	52.7	95.5
Working as labourer/family farm	21.1	100.0	40.0	—	—	81.8	33.1	42.1	58.3	39.5	31.3	93.9	36.4	50.0	100.0
Salaried/paid job	28.6	—	60.0	10.0	—	50.0	46.2	66.7	85.7	50.0	50.0	100.0	40.0	50.0	100.0
Migratory Status of Husband															
Non-migrant	16.8	—	62.0	9.0	76.9	35.1	53.3	46.6	53.1	59.0	48.6	89.0	45.3	45.8	100.0
Migrant	20.8	33.3	52.6	21.7	92.3	56.6	54.7	53.8	65.1	64.3	52.8	95.0	33.3	—	100.0
Exposure to Mass Media															
Yes	17.4	57.1	67.5	8.0	75.0	46.5	33.0	55.0	63.7	36.2	52.1	93.8	15.3	52.2	96.0
No	19.5	—	21.1	5.3	88.0	39.4	31.7	53.8	50.0	15.4	—	72.7	—	—	—
Total (N)	**19.3 (398)**	**57.1 (77)**	**64.8 (321)**	**7.5 (389)**	**86.2 (29)**	**45.1 (357)**	**32.9 (489)**	**54.9 (164)**	**62.6 (334)**	**35.6 (416)**	**51.4 (148)**	**92.9 (268)**	**15.3 (439)**	**52.2 (67)**	**95.7 (372)**

Note: 1. Ever been tested for HIV. 2. Tested in the last 12 months. 3. Knowing at least one place for HIV testing.

Figure 3.5

HIV testing among young women and men in the last 12 months prior to endline survey

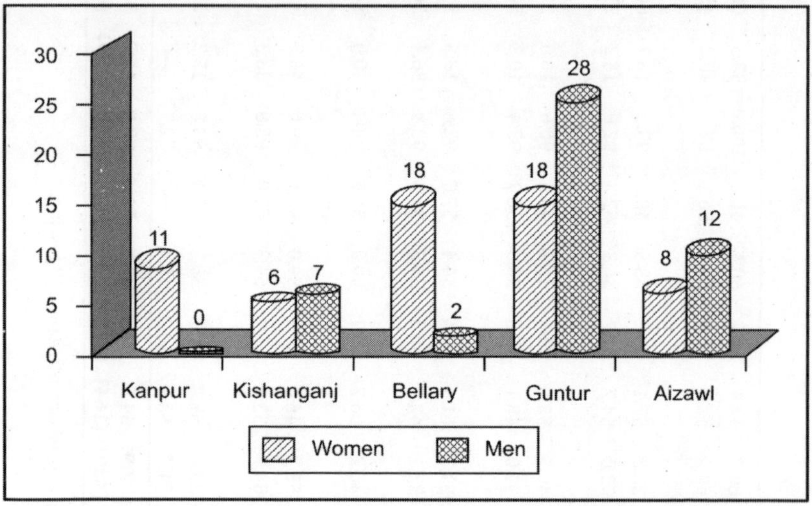

A substantial proportion of young men and young women who had never been tested for HIV know at least one place where HIV testing is done. Among young women the proportion knowing of a place ranges from 45 per cent in Kishanganj to 96 per cent in Aizawl. In the case of young men, it ranges from 28 per cent in Bellary to 96 per cent in Guntur. Young women aged 17–20, educated (10 years and above), unmarried, non-CBO members and those exposed to media are more likely to know of a place for HIV test in all the districts. Unlike other districts, in Aizawl, young women aged 21–24, illiterates, salaried and labourers and members of CBOs have better knowledge of a place for HIV test. Among young men knowledge of at least one place for HIV test varies across the districts.

Apparently, it seems that despite a substantial proportion of youth knowing of at least one place for HIV test, very few young men and young women reported ever having taken such a test. Even a larger proportion of young women than young men reported ever been tested for HIV, except in Aizawl and Kishanganj. One-third of the young women in Bellary, 36 per cent in Guntur, 19 per cent in Kanpur, 15 per cent in Aizawl and 8 per cent in Kishanganj have ever been tested for HIV. The pattern of HIV testing in the last 12 months prior to the survey reveals that 18 per cent of young women in each of Bellary and Guntur,

Table 3.8

Percentage of men aged 15–29 who reported they had ever tested for HIV and were tested in the last 12 months, and among those who were never tested for HIV, those knowing at least one place for HIV testing by selected background characteristics in CHARCA districts

	Kanpur			Kishanganj			Bellary			Guntur			Aizawl		
	1	2	3	1	2	3	1	2	3	1	2	3	1	2	3
Age (completed years)															
20 and below	0.7	100	49.3	5.3	100	79.8	5.0	20	29.2	21.4	93.3	98.2	25.0	39.1	95.2
20+	1.8	0.0	60.2	12	68.4	82.9	6.2	54.5	27.5	38.9	82.1	94.3	49	29.8	82.6
Marital Status															
Married	1.6	0.0	59.3	11	75.0	81.4	5.6	57.1	18.5	36.1	83.7	93.9	40	21.4	95.2
Unmarried	1.0	50	52.3	8.3	75.0	81.9	5.9	33.3	36.1	18.5	86.4	98.3	36.9	35.7	82.6
Education															
Illiterate	0.0	—	66.7	5.1	66.7	66.7	4.4	100	18.5	—	—	—	—	—	—
<5 years complete	0.0	—	33.3	5.3	100	66.7	4.0	0.0	16.7	50.0	85.7	100	0.0	—	—
5–7 years complete	2.9	100	39.4	9.3	100	83	0.0	—	22	30.4	85.7	91.7	—	—	—
8–9 years complete	0.0	—	61.0	9.8	100	86	3.2	0.0	13.3	44.4	87.5	100	7.7	100	91.7
10 years and above	1.9	0.0	57.2	13.6	54.5	94.2	10.0	36.4	44.4	30.2	86.2	98.5	40	31.9	85
Place of Residence															
Urban	—	—	—	—	—	—	5.9	100	43.8	38.3	87.0	94.6	38.5	32.1	85.2
Rural	1.3	100	55.1	9.4	75	81.7	5.7	40	27.1	31.2	83.3	96.2	34.7	35.3	84.4

Cont'd...

...Cont'd

Membership in CBOs/NGOs															
Yes	0.0	—	100	13	100	89.5	12.5	100	100	47.6	80	100	40.4	32.9	88
No	1.2	100	82.1	12.8	60	87.9	5.2	33.3	45.5	36.0	87.5	100	0.0	—	58.3
Occupation															
Students/not working	1.0	00	55.6	8.5	80	87	8.3	20	49.1	22.4	90.9	97.4	27.3	44.4	84.5
Working as labourer/family farm	0.6	100	49.1	5.0	66.7	84	4.7	55.6	23.8	36.0	82.0	95.5	46.9	37.5	84
Salaried/paid job	5.1	0.0	81.1	17.6	76.9	73.3	6.9	50	14.8	38.5	90.0	93.8	52.8	10.5	88.2
Migratory Status of Husband															
Non-migrant	0.0	—	56.7	8.8	71.4	78.7	3.6	57.1	22.3	39.2	84.3	94.9	53.2	25.6	83.2
Migrant	7.1	100	46.2	15.6	80.0	88.9	16.7	50	25	25.7	77.8	96.2	0.0	25.6	100
Exposure to Mass Media															
Yes	1.3	—	55.1	9.9	75	82.2	5.7	43.8	30.6	33.2	84.5	95.7	37.5	32.9	85.0
No	—	—	50	—	—	72.7	—	—	7.1	—	—	100*	—	—	—
Total (N)	**1.2* (322)**	**25* (1)**	**55.1 (316)**	**9.4 (254)**	**75 (24)**	**81.7 (224)**	**5.7 (317)**	**43.8 (16)**	**28.1 (263)**	**33.2 (214)**	**84.5 (71)**	**95.8 (143)**	**37.5 (184)**	**32.9 (70)**	**85.1 (114)**

* Less than five cases.

Note: 1. Ever been tested for HIV. 2. Tested in the last 12 months. 3. Knowing at least one place for HIV testing.

11 per cent in Kanpur, 8 per cent in Aizawl and 6 per cent in Kishanganj were tested in the last 12 months (Figure 3.5). The corresponding figures for young men are 2.4 per cent in Bellary, 28 per cent in Guntur, 0.3 per cent in Kanpur, 12 per cent in Aizawl and 7 per cent in Kishanganj. One can understand the extent of efforts made by CHARCA peer educators when we compare the above figures with the 2005–06 NFHS-3 national level estimates of HIV testing among youth in India.

'... in our village most of the people are aware of STIs/ HIV and other infections. This level of awareness has been seen in past few years due to several camps and awareness programmes. For example, awareness camps organized by ICDS and other CBOs/NGOs, supported by village panchayats have increased the awareness of STIs and HIV/AIDS in this community ...'

—Man KI, Guntur

'... the health camps are often organized in our village where doctors come to talk on healthy life and many times to check health too. These camps not only provide a treatment opportunity but also make the villagers aware regarding issues of healthcare including HIV prevention ...'

—Woman KI, Kanpur

'... in our time we were not knowing this much about health issues ... the young people are more aware than us. They are attending the meetings and other programmes organized by organizations in our village from time to time. Discussing with them clear many doubts regarding HIV and other health problems ...'

—Man KI, Bellary

'... earlier people of the village were not talking about HIV. They were scared of talking even in public, now they don't hesitate to advice others about the preventive measure of HIV ... even most of them know about the testing and many are going for it ...'

—Peer educator, FGD, Aizawl

'... there are many women who don't know to write except their names and few words ... still they are aware about reproductive health problems, HIV/AIDS and other sexual health issues. The awareness programme and the message is acting so effectively among the women in this community that it can be seen from the growing number of participants in weekly meetings organized in the village and the level of discussion happens there ...'

—Woman's FGD, Kishanganj

NFHS-3 estimates for the HIV testing among youth show 2.6 per cent among women aged 15–24 and 1.2 per cent among young men below age 25. Thus, barring young men in Kanpur, the levels of prevalence of HIV testing among young women as well as young men in the different districts reflects at the achievements of CHARCA in addressing the issues of stigma and discrimination and emphasizing the need for testing, which is a priority area in the NACP-III in the country.

Overall the level of awareness has increased substantially among young men and young women in all the districts and misconceptions have reduced considerably. More insights about the improvement in awareness of STIs and HIV/AIDS among young people have been mentioned by local key informants and focus groups in the districts. From their views and opinions it is clear that many factors are responsible for the increase in awareness and knowledge about HIV/STIs.

Attitude towards people living with HIV/AIDS

The attitudes of people in the community towards HIV positive people have been associated with the increasing prevalence of HIV/AIDS. Increasingly the HIV positive people also face stigma and discrimination which make care and treatment more difficult. A series of questions were asked to young men and women regarding their attitudes towards the persons infected with HIV/AIDS. Three of the important responses were taken into consideration to indicate a positive attitude towards HIV positive people. Tables 3.9 and 3.10 present the data in this regard. It is found that a majority of male and female respondents have positive attitudes towards people living with HIV/AIDS. It is heartening to note that the proportion with positive attitudes has increased substantially in most districts when compared to the baseline survey.

A majority of the young women reported that HIV positive people should not be terminated from jobs and this proportion has increased over time (Table 3.9). Compared to the baseline results, the proportion with negative attitudes has declined sharply in all the states but is more prominent in Kanpur (from 92% to 12%) and Aizawl (from 83% to 1%). The decline is also substantial in Kishanganj (from 76% to 30%), Guntur (from 68% to 21%) and Bellary (from 45% to 10%). A mixed but positive change in the attitudes is also reflected when asked about HIV positive persons mixing with others or visiting public places in most districts. The decline over the period has not been as sharp as in the case of termination from jobs. Interestingly, in Bellary and Kishanganj, the proportion has shown an increase, from 38 per cent to

77 per cent and from 15 per cent to 23 per cent respectively. Despite increased awareness about HIV/AIDS, the presence of stigma and discrimination among some sections of the people in the community in every district is clearly reflected. The variation reflected in the attitude has a potential policy implication and calls for a strategic change in awareness campaigns, which is also mentioned by some key persons in the qualitative data gathering.

Table 3.9

Attitudes of women towards people living with HIV/AIDS (%)

Attitudes	*Kanpur**	*Kishanganj*		*Bellary*		*Guntur*		*Aizawl*	
	EL	*BL*	*EL*	*BL*	*EL*	*BL*	*EL*	*BL*	*EL*
HIV+ person should be terminated from services if in job	**11.6**	76.3	**29.6**	44.8	**10.2**	67.5	**20.7**	82.6	**1.1**
HIV+ person should not mix up with others or visit public places	**5.0**	14.8	**22.9**	37.9	**77.1**	56.6	**2.7**	73.6	**44.2**
HIV+ person should be provided with specialized healthcare	**94.5**	87.1	**75.8**	80.4	**30.7**	80.5	**98.8**	98.0	**99.8**
Total Women	**398**	539	**389**	488	**498**	472	**415**	471	**439**

* Information from the baseline survey is not presented due to change in intervention after the baseline survey.

Compared to the baseline results, most young women who opine that HIV positive persons need special healthcare, range from 31 per cent in Bellary to 100 per cent in Aizawl. Despite the high proportion, in fact, in three districts, namely, Kanpur, Kishanganj and Bellary, the proportion has shown a decline, with nearly 50 percentage points in Bellary. Such a mixed reaction is also found in different communities in the field through key informants and focus groups.

The panel data on attitudes of women towards people living with HIV/AIDS reveals that the proportion of respondents reporting that HIV positive persons should not be terminated from service has increased in the districts of Guntur, Aizawl and Bellary over the baseline survey. In the case whether an HIV positive person should mix with people in public places, the proportion of respondents who responded in the affirmative has increased over the period. More than one-third young women in Bellary and Guntur feel that HIV positive persons should be provided with specialized healthcare. The proportion in Kishanganj is 17 per cent and in Kanpur 9 per cent. There

Table 3.10

Attitudes of men towards people living with HIV/AIDS (%)

Attitudes	*Kanpur**	*Kishanganj*		*Bellary*		*Guntur*		*Aizawl*	
	EL	*BL*	*EL*	*BL*	*EL*	*BL*	*EL*	*BL*	*EL*
HIV+ person should be terminated from services if in job	**11.3**	57.2	**10.3**	59.4	**30.8**	74.6	**50.9**	85.5	**3.3**
A HIV+ person should not mix up with others or visit public places	**5.3**	33.8	**12.3**	41	**54.8**	65.9	**97.7**	72.1	**2.7**
HIV+ person should be provided with specialized health care	**96.3**	81.7	**96.4**	84	**57.7**	92.8	**97.7**	98.6	**98.9**
Total Men	**322**	291	**328**	256	**279**	264	**214**	220	**184**

* Information from the baseline survey is not presented due to change in intervention after the baseline survey.

is thus a positive change in the perception of the women towards people living with HIV/AIDS in most of the states and it is mainly attributed to CHARCA intervention.

Young men were asked similar questions about their attitudes towards HIV positive persons. A significant proportion had responded in the affirmative so far as the termination from services of HIV positive persons is concerned in the baseline survey, ranging from 57 per cent in Kishanganj to 97 per cent in Kanpur. In the endline survey, the proportion has declined further in most districts, ranging from 3 per cent in Aizawl to 51 per cent in Guntur. Aizawl and Kanpur show more significant decline than other districts. Young men's attitude on 'HIV positive persons should mix with others or visit public places' and 'HIV positive persons should be provided with specialized healthcare' is similar to that of young women. In Bellary and Guntur more young men believe that HIV positive persons should mix with others or visit public places. In Guntur the proportion has increased from 66 per cent to 98 per cent and in Bellary from 41 per cent to 55 per cent in the endline survey. Besides, most young men still think that HIV positive persons need special care, but over the period the view has not changed much. Again Bellary and Kanpur show a decrease in the proportion of those who feel that HIV positive persons should be provided with specialized care.

In an analogous fashion the qualitative data also revealed that the attitudes towards the people leaving with HIV have changed over the time period. The long-term awareness programme regarding the preventive behaviour of HIV, gender sensitization and sexual health lessened the stigma attached with the notion of HIV/AIDS. The direct

> '... the misconception about HIV is reducing ... earlier we were not aware of the issue. So we used to believe in lots of stories we heard from different sources. Now things are getting clearer and we know how the HIV spreads and how not ... the fear about the HIV has been reduced, rather people are more aware of it.'
>
> —Man KI, Guntur
>
> '... health workers used to come to us and talk about HIV and other problems ... they tell us how it gets transmitted, and what are the misconceptions about spreading of HIV which was the main reason of outcasting the people with HIV ... now I don't get afraid of talking to any person with AIDS or even staying with him/her ...'
>
> —Woman KI, Kishanganj
>
> '... The most important contribution of CHARCA has been the networking of positive people. The networking and interaction with many other positive people have reduced our guilt and shown a new ray of hope in life ...'
>
> —PLWHA FGD, Kanpur
>
> '... From the last seven years I am positive ... in our house there is no problem ... they cooperate with me well and don't discriminate though earlier they had some problem in accepting me ... now they are encouraging me ... They also tell me not to go for work ... sometimes my mother-in-law used to comment that only because of me my husband got the infection ... but she is changing slowly ... nowadays she knows more about the disease and getting sensitized ...'
>
> —Woman PLWHA, Bellary
>
> '... things have changed a lot around our community. Now, there are instances where people go easy with people infected with HIV ... villagers trying to help the people with HIV at all possible levels. Even sometimes financially though the financial condition of villagers is not good ...'
>
> —Man KI, Aizawl
>
> '... people used to cooperate with them financially also... but some educated ones who are not aware of HIV hate them and treat them as untouchables. They think that they can be infected through HIV if they will see or eat or touch HIV infected person ...'
>
> —Peer educators, FGD, Kishanganj

thrusts of awareness about HIV transmission has effectively contributed in changing the attitude of young men and women across the five districts towards the people living with HIV. It has apparently appeared during FGDs with PLWHA (People Living with HIV/AIDS) across different states that in spite of implications of disclosures in terms of different forms of stigma in the family, community and society as a whole, there have been changes in the people's attitude towards HIV infected persons in the recent years. Now, it has been relatively easier to disclose HIV status and get benefits of different programmes and activities initiated by the government and other social organizations. Incidence of violence against women, especially wives of HIV positive men, have definitely declined in recent years.

In fact, this has happened due to increasing awareness among people over time and now the situation has changed and people do not blame the wife if a husband is detected as HIV positive. As a result, social acceptance of wives of HIV infected persons has improved in recent years. The credit for these attitudinal changes should be given to non-government organizations and other community-based programmes like CHARCA, which have continuously been motivating people not to discriminate those who are infected with HIV.

It is amply evident from the qualitative insights through KI interviews and FGDs that CHARCA has made a significant contribution in the life of HIV infected persons. The first and most important contribution of CHARCA has been the networking of positive people. Networking and interaction with other positive people has reduced our guilt and shown a new ray of hope in life. All subsequent support in terms of physical examination even by sending them to nearby cities, arrangements of ARTs, organization of different types of skill development programmes, ensuring economic empowerment of positive people who wanted to be self-dependent, providing job opportunity to work as outreach workers in the programmes and activities for PLWHA have made a significant contribution in the lives of positive people in CHARCA districts. It is the CHARCA programme which has always stood with the group of positive people and raised the issues of their rights, whenever there is some crisis in terms of medication and/or stigma and discrimination.

Summary of findings and conclusions

- Awareness about HIV/AIDS has shown tremendous improvement in four of the five districts between the two surveys. A significant increase has also been observed in the level of awareness among young women in the panel sample, which may be attributed to the range of programmes and activities organized under the CHARCA intervention.

- The level of awareness about HIV/AIDS among young men and women appears to depend more on social characteristics such as education and exposure to media. However, a significant increase in HIV/AIDS awareness among those exposed to media in all the districts except Kanpur can be attributed to the macro- and micro-level programmes and activities organized under the CHARCA intervention. NGOs/CBOs and health professionals have also emerged main as the sources of information in the endline survey.
- A large proportion of the young men and women perceive that using condom consistently during each sexual intercourse can prevent HIV/AIDS. The change in the perception is also quite significant in the panel sample. More young women aged 13–16, illiterate, unmarried, rural residents, working as labourers and not exposed to media do not perceive and are likely to be less aware that consistent use of condom during each sexual intercourse can protect a person against HIV. However, the gap in such awareness among young women is found to be wider by exposure to media and education, especially in Kanpur and Kishanganj.
- Compared to the baseline results, each district records a substantial increase in young men's awareness about condom use as protection against STIs or HIV/AIDS. The importance of condom, despite its low use in all the districts, is also expressed strongly by many young men.
- In three of the five districts (viz., Kishanganj, Bellary and Guntur) there has been a substantial increase over the baseline survey in the proportion of young men knowing about other preventive measures such as 'checking blood prior to transfusion', 'sterilizing needles and syringes for injections', 'avoiding sex with CSWs' and 'sex with only one partner', in all the districts, barring Kanpur.
- The perception young women have about 'sex with only one partner' as a preventive measure varies by their background characteristics across the five districts. As mentioned in other cases earlier, Aizawl (and to a certain extent in Guntur) shows no variation by different characteristics as the awareness level is universal. In other districts, the gap is more prominent by education and exposure to media among young women.

- A drastic decrease in the proportion of young women with at least one misconception about HIV/AIDS in all the districts except in Kishanganj is consistent with the extent of increase in awareness over the CHARCA intervention period. However, young women who are more likely to have at least one misconception about acquiring HIV/AIDS than others are in the age group 21–24, illiterates, non-members of CBOs/NGOs, and those with no exposure to media. Therefore, any community-based intervention should target these groups through innovative approaches reinforcing these messages on a constant basis.
- The endline survey reveals a considerably higher prevalence of HIV testing among youth in the CHARCA districts than the rates reported by other recent studies. More young women than men reported that they had ever been tested for HIV, except in Aizawl and Kishanganj. One-third of the young women in Bellary as well as in Guntur, 19 per cent in Kanpur, 15 per cent in Aizawl and 8 per cent in Kishanganj have ever been tested for HIV. This clearly brings out the outcomes of concerted efforts of CHARCA at minimizing the stigma associated with HIV and motivating people to use IVCTC services.
- A major proportion of young men and women reported positive attitudes towards people living with HIV/AIDS, and these proportions have increased over the last three years. Qualitative insights on attitude towards PLWHA affirm a change in people's attitude towards PLWHA with reduction in stigma and discrimination and a very conducive environment for testing and disclosure of HIV status. The contribution of CHARCA functionaries in improving the quality of life of PLWHA cuts across all the five districts where the major contributions have been reported in developing a network of positive people, opening of drop-in centres, arranging for ARTs and testing of CD4 counts and treatment of opportunistic infections.

4

Reproductive, Sexual and Women's Rights

For the success of reproductive health programmes, there is a need to recognize their multidimensional character and look beyond the delivery of maternal and child health (MCH) or family planning services. The reproductive health concept is a 'rights-oriented as well as health-oriented', which 'recognizes that sexual as well as reproductive health and rights are vital elements of physical and emotional well-being' (Dixon-Mueller, 1993; Germain and Ordway, 1989; POA-ICPD, 1994). Further, the POA of ICPD specifies that men and women must have the right to be informed and have access to safe, effective, affordable and acceptable methods of their choice for the regulation of fertility, as well as access to healthcare for safe pregnancy and childbirth (UN/POA, 1994).

In a male-dominated society, generally issues related to attitudes and behaviours about sexuality and particularly about female autonomy in health matters are important concerns. For instance, the fact that women in India seek husband's permission to obtain some basic health needs reflects the community perception about women's autonomy and status. Similarly, the number of women using contraceptive methods of their choice is an important reflection of the community's perspective on roles related to reproductive and sexual rights.

In the present study, to assess young women's attitudes towards and perceptions of reproductive and sexual rights, a series of questions were asked about their perceptions on the decisions to be taken on matters concerning their reproductive health and sexual behaviours. This chapter deals with the women's responses in these matters.

Women seeking husband's permission for health-related matters and to attend CBO/NGO meetings

Tables 4.1 and 4.2 present the women's actual behaviour as well as perceptions of rights-related issues that reflect the extent of independence and participation of women in community activities. Table 4.1 shows the proportion of women who do not have to seek husband's permission for their own health-related matters. The data reveals a decline in the proportion of such women in all the districts, except in Kishanganj. The decline is more prominent in Guntur (1% in endline from 10% in baseline). A similar trend is observed in the use of contraceptives of their choice in all the districts. However, the decline is much higher than in the case of healthcare services for self. Except in Bellary, there has been a decline in the proportion of women who do not seek husband's permission to use contraceptives. In Bellary, one-fourth of the women do not seek husband's permission to use contraceptive of their choice, followed by Kishanganj (19%) and Kanpur (7%). It implies that women have fewer roles in decision-making and they still require their husband's permission to avail of basic healthcare services.

Table 4.1

Percentage of women who do not seek husband's permission/decision for their health-related matters

Health-related matters	*Kanpur**	*Kishanganj*		*Bellary*		*Guntur*		*Aizawl*	
	EL	*BL*	*EL*	*BL*	*EL*	*BL*	*EL*	*BL*	*EL*
To seek healthcare services for self	**3.6**	7.3	**17.7**	2.5	**0.8**	10.1	**1.3**	4.9	**0.0**
To use contraceptive of her choice	**7.1**	40.6	**19.4**	1.8	**24.9**	18.1	**2.6**	33.3	**5.6**
Total Women	**169**	234	**248**	284	**261**	249	**235**	81	**72**

* Information from the baseline survey is not presented due to change in intervention after the baseline survey.

The panel data also indicate an increase in the proportion of women who do not require husband's permission to seek healthcare services for self when compared to the baseline survey in the districts of Bellary and Kishanganj. On contraceptive autonomy as well, more women do not seek husband's permission to use contraceptives of their choice in the districts of Kanpur and Aizawl than in other districts. This positive change in the autonomy of females has occurred due to the intervention of CHARCA programme.

From women's responses, lack of inter-spousal communication among married couples is indicated in most of the districts. The decision on number of children as well as the choice of contraceptive methods is still determined by the husbands in a majority of cases.

Table 4.2 presents the perceptions of females regarding the need for permission to attend Mahila Mandal/CBO/NGO meetings. One-fourth of the women in Kishanganj, followed by Bellary (17%) and Kanpur (8%), perceive that the wife does not need husband's permission to participate in the Mahila Mandal/CBO/NGO meetings. There has been a consistent decline in the proportion of women who perceive that wife does not need husband's permission to participate in the activities of Mahila Mandals/CBOs/NGOs in all the districts excepting Bellary, in comparison to the baseline survey. It is quite interesting to note that across all the districts, the proportion of young men who perceive that wife does not need husband's permission to participate in such community meetings is quite high compared to women. The highest proportion is reported in Bellary (46%), followed by Guntur (23%) and Kanpur (20%). The findings thus reflect that women can take care of their health needs without seeking prior permission from their husbands.

Table 4.2

Percentage of women who perceived wife does not need husband's permission/ decision to participate in the activities in Mahila Mandals/CBOs/NGOs

Sex	*Kanpur**	*Kishanganj*		*Bellary*		*Guntur*		*Aizawl*	
	EL	*BL*	*EL*	*BL*	*EL*	*BL*	*EL*	*BL*	*EL*
Male	19.8 (126)	22.2 (120)	13.3 (150)	11.7 (120)	46.4 (179)	11.2 (127)	23 (131)	8.8 (49)	17.1 (35)
Female	8.3 (169)	76.5 (234)	25.4 (248)	0.4 (284)	17.2 (261)	17.5 (249)	1.3 (235)	18.8 (81)	6.9 (72)

* Information from the baseline survey is not presented due to change in intervention after the baseline survey.

The panel data on autonomy of women in terms of membership of community-based organizations show an increase in the proportion of women who do not require husband's permission to participate in Mahila Mandals/CBOs/NGOs in the districts of Kanpur, Guntur and Aizawl compared to the baseline survey. The impact of intervention is clearly visible in terms of enhancing female autonomy in most of the project districts.

Information on men's perception regarding women's contraceptive choice was collected and the results are presented by their socio-economic and demographic background like education, place of residence, membership in CBOs/NGOs, occupation, age, marital status, etc. in Table 4.3. A majority of the young men in all the districts perceive that a wife can choose contraception of her choice. There is considerable increase in the proportion of such men who recognize that the decision about the contraceptive to be used should largely depend on wives. This proportion is higher among young men aged 20 or less than among aged 20 or above, ranging from 65 per cent in Kanpur to 100 per cent in Guntur. The substantial increase in men's perception indicated over the baseline survey in 2004 can be attributed to macro-level programmes and activities organized under the CHARCA intervention to enhance male participation in women's programme by creating an enabling environment.

Regarding marital status, a majority of unmarried young men feel that the wives can use contraceptives of their choice and this proportion has increased in comparison with the baseline survey in all the districts except Aizawl, where it has declined marginally. Education of men is an important factor which influences perception of female autonomy in the use of contraceptive methods. Table 4.3 shows that about two-thirds of illiterate young men in Kanpur, Kishanganj and Bellary perceive that a wife can use contraceptive of her choice. The proportion increases sharply for those having 10 or more years and above of education ranging from 71 per cent in Aizawl and Kanpur to over 90 per cent in Bellary and Guntur.

The survey also reveals that membership in CBOs/NGOs reflects positive perceptions as such members are more likely to accept their wife's choice and use of contraceptive methods in most districts except Aizawl. Young men's characteristics, such as occupation, exposure to media or migrant status, do not reflect much variation in perception about use and choice of contraceptives by their wives.

Table 4.3

Percentage of young male perceiving that a wife can choose contraception of her choice

Background characteristics	*Kanpur**	*Kishanganj*		*Bellary*		*Guntur*		*Aizawl*	
	EL	*BL*	*EL*	*BL*	*EL*	*BL*	*EL*	*BL*	*EL*
Age (completed years)									
20 and below	**65.1**	47.2	**69.2**	36.8	**93.5**	37.4	**100**	73.9	**73.9**
20+	**62.9**	39.4	**65.5**	38.0	**90.2**	30.5	**95.1**	74.3	**67.7**
Marital Status									
Married	**62.7**	44.3	**61.4**	37.5	**88.4**	37.1	**95.4**	74.3	**77.1**
Unmarried	**64.8**	40.3	**71.5**	37.3	**93.9**	29.9	**98.1**	74.5	**69.1**
Education									
Illiterate	**66.7**	35.4	**65.7**	34.0	**84.7**	14.3†	**0.0**	0.0	**0.0**
<5 years complete	**66.7**	44.1	**60.9**	25.7	**85.7**	46.2	**100**	66.7	**100**
5–7 years complete	**63.9**	53.8	**58.1**	29.7	**92.7**	23.1	**97.1**	76.5	**0.0**
8–9 years complete	**52.0**	45.2	**67.4**	37.8	**97.1**	42.9	**100**	74.1	**61.5**
10 and above	**71.0**	48.6	**75.9**	47.4	**95.6**	36.8	**95.8**	73.4	**71.2**
Membership in CBOs/NGOs									
Yes	**50**	75.0†	**80**	47.1	**62.5**	34.4	**100**	74.6	**69.0**
No	**42**	40.0†	**70.7**	39.0	**96.7**	48.5	**94.4**	15.0†	**100**
Occupation									
Student/not working	**68**	48.6	**70.1**	58.3	**95.4**	30.6	**100**	67.9	**78.8**
Working as labourer/family farm	**66.3**	41.4	**63.1**	32.0	**89.6**	35.9	**96.4**	71.4	**59.2**
Salaried/paid job	**42.6**	45.2	**70.8**	37.6	**96.8**	23.9	**92.3**	87.8	**63.9**
Total (N)	**64.0 (322)**	42.1 (291)	**66.9 (328)**	37.5 (256)	**91.5 (317)**	33.1 (264)	**96.7 (214)**	74.0 (220)	**70.7 (184)**

* Information from the baseline survey is not presented due to change in intervention after the baseline survey.

† Less than five cases.

The qualitative insights on the women's rights and autonomy are also parallel with the survey findings. Women status in terms of independency in the choice of contraceptives and mobility still needs intervention across the five districts, though the scenario has improved in some of the districts. Changing the age-old male dominance and normalization of the patriarchy even among the women is definitely a challenge before any programme and action. However, it is a positive sign for sure that the women in a largely rural Indian set-up have started talking about and reacting to the issues

'... I know a woman in our village who is having problems regarding her sexual life with her husband ... she wants her husband to use condom instead of herself taking oral pills as she is having vomiting and weakness after taking oral pills regularly. But her husband does not use as he argues that using condom does not give satisfaction during sex ...'

—Woman KI, Bellary

'... one of my friends is suffering from mistreatment her from in-laws frequently ... I have tried to convince my friend to speak up at home if some wrong things happen ... I know it is difficult but unless we open up our mouth, how they will know that we can speak? if they are not sensitive enough to recognize our rights we must demand it ...'

—Woman FGD, Kanpur

'... initially my family members were getting angry when I used go for meeting with CHARCA, later on I used to come and discuss about healthcare issues and healthy life in my family they gradually began to accept my advices. Now, they realize I am going for a good cause and not raising any issue regarding my meeting attendance ...'

—Woman KI, Guntur

'... the participation of married women in health *melas* and other meetings has increased over period of time ... initially we used escort them, we have to convince their husbands that it will be beneficial for their own family then only they let their wives take part in our meetings ... but now when they see that their wives are getting the attention of fellow women in the villages as other seek advice regarding health and other matters to their wives they started encouraging their wives' participation ... now most of the women come on their own. Even if we organize zonal meetings far from the village.'

—Peer educator, FGD, Kishanganj

'... women have also right to live their life, move freely. They have every right to take their decisions about issues in their life. It is not good to impose men's decision on them unnecessarily ... I was behaving like others few years before unless the programme people talked to me and saw the messages, then I felt how my wife has suffered. I have changed in my life ...'

—Young man, FGD, Aizawl

related to their rights at different levels. Further, in some places young women have tried to bring a change in their personal lives.

Perception of young men towards sexual rights of women

Men's attitude towards sexual rights of women is an important indicator for the better understanding of women's health problems. Table 4.4 reveals that a majority of men agree that women have the right to enjoy sex and the responses vary from 82 per cent to 99 per cent in the baseline survey. A similar pattern is observed in the endline survey, where almost all the men agree that women have the right to enjoy sex, ranging above 90 per cent with the highest in Aizawl (99%).

Table 4.4

Perception of young men towards the sexual right of women in the five CHARCA districts (%)

Perception towards women sexual rights	*Kanpur**	*Kishanganj*		*Bellary*		*Guntur*		*Aizawl*	
	EL	*BL*	*EL*	*BL*	*EL*	*BL*	*EL*	*BL*	*EL*
A wife has a right to enjoy sex	**96.6**	93.7	**92.1**	82.4	**91.2**	99.2	**95.3**	98.1	**98.9**
A wife can say 'no' to husband if she does not want sex	**98.8**	90.7	**93.3**	88.3	**83.9**	97.3	**97.2**	97.3	**99.5**
A wife should not accept her husband's extra-marital relations	**98.8**	87.5	**96.3**	66.8	**66.6**	96.9	**78**	96.9	**100**
Total	**322**	291	**328**	256	**317**	264	**214**	220	**184**

* Information from the baseline survey is not presented due to change in intervention after the baseline survey.

A positive response is reported across all the districts when men are asked whether 'a wife can say no to husband if she does not want sex'. In all the districts around 88 to 100 per cent responded positively or agreed that a wife can say no to husband if she does not want sex without much variation across the states. In the endline survey, except in Bellary and Guntur, where there is a slight decline in men reporting that a wife can say no to her husband when she does not want sex, in the other districts there is an increase in the proportion of men agreeing with the same. Except in Bellary, more than 90 per cent of men in the CHARCA districts perceive or have a positive attitude towards women's sexual rights.

There are variations in the responses when young men were asked 'whether a wife should not accept husband's extra-marital relationship'. In the baseline survey it was 67 per cent in Bellary. In the remaining states 88 to 97 per cent of the men agreed that women should not accept their husband's extra-marital relationship. In the endline survey, Bellary remains the same with 67 per cent. In Aizawl all men (100%) agreed that women should not accept their husband's extra-marital relationship.

In both the baseline and endline surveys, as shown in Table 4.4, across all the districts, a majority of the men agreed that women have the right to enjoy sex and there was not much variation in their responses. To understand the possible variations, if any, in matters of reproductive right in various categories of sub-population across the districts, perception of men that a wife has the right to enjoy sex is examined by some selected background characteristics.

Table 4.5 shows that in the baseline survey no uniform variation is observed across all the districts within various categories of sub-populations. Young men aged more than 20 years are more favourable in their attitude towards women's reproductive and sexual rights in Bellary (86%) than in other districts.

Regarding their opinion by marital status, it is found that unmarried men have a comparatively favourable attitude towards women's reproductive rights in Kishanganj and Bellary. Similarly, literate men are more likely to express a positive attitude in matters of sexual rights than the illiterate men.

The endline survey shows that except in Guntur, there is an increase in the perception of men that a wife has right to enjoy sex with increase in age. More men aged 20 and above opine that women has the right to enjoy sex as in Aizawl (100%) and Kanpur (96.5%) compared to other districts. In Guntur, men aged 20 and below are more favourable (97%) in their attitude towards women's right to enjoy sex. According to marital status, a higher proportion of married men in Aizawl (100%), Kishanganj (95.3%) and Bellary (93%) perceive that a wife has the right to enjoy sex compared to the unmarried young men. Despite a minor differences, more unmarried young men in Kanpur (97%) and Guntur (96%) also perceive that women have reproductive and sexual rights. Young men's educational level also, except in Kanpur and Kishanganj, reflects a positive attitude towards women's sexual rights than the illiterates. Similarly, a higher proportion of men, who are members of CBOs/NGOs, doing salaried/paid job, and are non-migrants, discern that a wife has the right to enjoy sex. Exposure to media does not seem to have any impact on the perception of young men regarding sexual rights.

Table 4.5

Percentage of young men perceiving that a wife has right to enjoy sex by background characteristics

Background characteristics	*Kanpur**	*Kishanganj*		*Bellary*		*Guntur*		*Aizawl*	
	EL	*BL*	*EL*	*BL*	*EL*	*BL*	*EL*	*BL*	*EL*
Age (completed years)									
20 and below	**96.7**	96.8	**93.2**	77.4	**87.0**	100.0	**97.0**	100	**98.9**
20+	**96.5**	91.6	**94.1**	86.0	**93.8**	99.4	**94.4**	96.0	**100.0**
Marital Status									
Married	**96**	89.2	**95.3**	81.7	**92.8**	100.0	**94.7**	98	**100.0**
Unmarried	**96.9**	97.1	**92.4**	83.1	**89.9**	99.1	**96.3**	98.2	**99.3**
Education									
Illiterate	**100.0**	91.9	**94.1**	75.0	**87.1**	100.0	**0.0**	0.0	**0.0**
<5 years complete	**95.2**	95.6	**96.0**	80.0	**89.3**	100.0	**100.0**	88.9	**100.0**
5–7 years complete	**94.4**	97.4	**95.2**	86.5	**90.9**	100.0	**94.2**	97.1	**0.0**
8–9 years complete	**98.0**	95.2	**93.5**	89.2	**91.4**	100.0	**100.0**	98.8	**100.0**
10 and above	**96.3**	88.6	**92.0**	82.5	**94.7**	99.2	**94.8**	98.9	**99.4**
Membership in CBOs/NGOs									
Yes	**100.0**	100.0	**96.0**	82.4	**100.0**	100.0	**100.0**	98.1	**99.4**
No	**96.8**	80.0	**95.2**	84.6	**91.7**	100.0	**92.1**	100.0	**100.0**
Occupation									
Student/not working	**97**	97.3	**94.0**	79.2	**92.3**	98.0	**98**	100.0	**100.0**
Working as labourer/family farm	**95.5**	94.6	**93**	83.1	**89.6**	100.0	**94.1**	96.7	**98**
Salaried/paid job	**100**	83.9	**94.6**	83.3	**100**	100.0	**96.2**	98.0	**100.0**
Total (N)	**96.6 (322)**	**93.7 (291)**	**92.1 (328)**	**82.4 (256)**	**91.2 (317)**	**99.6 (263)**	**95.3 (214)**	**98.2 (220)**	**99.3 (184)**

* Information from the baseline survey is not presented due to change in intervention after the baseline survey.

Despite the universal perception among young males that a wife has the right to enjoy sex, mere positive perception is not sufficient unless it is translated into positive action of respecting women. Views expressed during Key Informant (KI) interviews and Focus Group Discussions (FGDs) reveal the existence of male dominance, status hierarchy and unequal power relations, which highlight the vulnerability of women and their inability to exercise their rights. These views suggest a need to strategically bring about changes in perceptions and attitudes of men, women and society as a whole.

Sexual rights of women

Regarding perceptions about sexual rights, women were asked, 'Do you think a woman has the right to refuse sex?' For the purpose of analysis to capture and reflect women's sexual rights, the responses 'agree' and 'somewhat agree' were merged to connote 'agree'. It was finally dichotomized as women who agreed and those who disagreed. Disagreement with the statement is considered as inability to refuse sex.

Table 4.6 shows that only few women could refuse sex, which varies from 17 per cent in Bellary to less than 1 per cent in Aizawl. The proportion is high in Bellary, followed by Kishanganj (10%), which also reflects the low status of women and female subjugation in Bellary and Kishanganj compared to women in Aizawl.

The bivariate table (Table 4.6) reveals that in Bellary and Kishanganj the inability to refuse sex by women decreases with an increase in age, whereas in Kanpur and Guntur it increases with an increase in age. More married women reported their inability to refuse sex in Kanpur (5%) and Kishanganj (10%) compared to unmarried young women (2% and 9% respectively). However, in Bellary (20%), Guntur and Aizawl (less than 1%), more unmarried women report incapable of refusing sex compared to the married women. Literacy of women has a positive impact on the ability of refusal of sex. Except in Guntur, the illiterate women are more unlikely to refuse sex compared to literate women. Membership in CBOs/NGOs does not seem to have an impact on the ability to refuse sex in all the CHARCA districts, except in Kishanganj where more women who are non-members in CBO/NGO reported not being able to refuse sex (33%).

Surprisingly, across all the districts, exposure to media shows a low impact. Despite exposure to media, women are found not empowered to refuse sex. This finding contradicts with the baseline findings where mass media really showed a positive impact on refusal of unwanted sexual encounters. In general, except for Aizawl, compared to homemakers/housewives, working women are less likely to refuse sex. Women who are engaged as labourers or who work in the family farm seem to have lesser ability to refuse sex in Bellary and Kanpur, and salaried/paid job women in Kishanganj have lesser ability to refuse sex. By husband's migratory status also, as found in Kishanganj and Bellary, women are not capable to refuse sex when they do not want to.

Overall, women's inability to refuse sex decreased from 46 per cent to 10 per cent in Kishanganj, 51 per cent to 17 per cent in Bellary, 42 per cent to 0.5 per cent in Guntur and 6 per cent to 0.2 per cent in Aizawl. The panel data (Figure 4.1) also presents the overall decline in proportion of women who do not have ability to refuse sex.

Table 4.6

Percentage of young women who don't have ability to refuse sex if they do not want to by selected characteristics in CHARCA districts

Background characteristics	*Kanpur**	*Kishanganj*		*Bellary*		*Guntur*		*Aizawl*	
	EL	*BL*	*EL*	*BL*	*EL*	*BL*	*EL*	*BL*	*EL*
Age (completed years)									
13–16	**2.0**	25.8	**13.6**	22.4	**23.6**	27.3	**0.0**	2.2†	**0.9**
17–20	**2.1**	43.8	**10.4**	54.2	**15.9**	46.8	**0.0**	7.4	**0.0**
21–24	**5.6**	69.9	**6.8**	72.3	**11.4**	49.2	**1.2**	6.9	**0.0**
Marital Status									
Married	**4.8**	76.4	**10.1**	71.5	**14.2**	57.1	**0.4**	10.7	**0.0**
Unmarried	**2.2**	22.5	**9.2**	20.4	**20.1**	24.5	**0.5**	4.7	**0.3**
Women's Education									
Illiterate	**2.2**	58.6	**10.0**	70.6	**17.3**	53.9	0.0	0.0	**0.0**
<5 years complete	**15.8**	49.2	**14.4**	60.8	**13.3**	76.0	**0.0**	11.8	**0.0**
5–7 years complete	**3.5**	32.7	**9.1**	46.2	**22.5**	43.7	**0.8**	6.0	**2.3**
8–9 years complete	**3.5**	21.8	**7.1**	29.9	**17.1**	30.4	**0.0**	4.9	**0.0**
10 years and above	**1.8**	34.7	**4.9**	26.7	**14.1**	31.4	**0.7**	5.9	**0.0**
Membership in CBOs/NGOs									
Yes	**5.9**	33.3	**13.0**	50	**23.7**	44.9	**1.1**	6.3	**0.0**
No	**3.2**	45.7	**33.3**	51.2	**18.3**	41.6	**0.0**	5.0	**1.7**
Women's Occupation									
Homemaker	**3.1**	43.9	**9.8**	41.6	**14.4**	37.2	**0.3**	5.4	**0.2**
Working as Labourer/family farm	**4.3**	78.9	**6.3**	64.7	**23**	48.8	**1.2**	9.8†	**0.0**
salaried/paid job	**0.0**	33.3†	**10.0**	65.4	**9.7**	61.5	**0.0**	5.3†	**0.0**
Migratory Status of Husband									
Non-migrant	**6.1**	44.4	**5.6**	51.3	**13.6**	42.1	**0.6**	5.3	**0.0**
Migrant	**0.0**	69.2	**21.4**	33.3†	**15.1**	50	**0.0**	0.0	**0.0**
Exposure to Mass Media									
Yes	**3.2**	40.1	**10.3**	47.7	**17.2**	38.8	**7.7**	5.8	**0.2**
No	**1.9**	64.5	**7.7**	82.6	**16.1**	59.2	**0.2**	0.0	**0.0**
Total (N)	**3.1**	45.6	**9.7**	51.2	**17.1**	42.1	**0.5**	5.7	**0.2**
	(494)	(539)	**(465)**	(467)	**(556)**	(472)	**(417)**	(471)	**(439)**

* Information from the baseline survey is not presented due to change in intervention after the baseline survey.

† Less than five cases.

The panel data (Figure 4.1) show a drastic decrease in the proportion of women who do not have ability to refuse sex. The change in the proportion of women who do not have the ability to refuse sex in the last three years (from baseline survey to endline survey) is more obvious in Aizawl. The proportion drops to zero from 79 per cent highlighting almost universal ability of women to refuse sex. Guntur and Kishanganj also show significant drop in the percentage of women who do not have the ability to refuse sex. The proportion decreases by 52 per cent in Guntur and 48 per cent in Kishanganj.

Figure 4.1

Proportion of women who do not have ability to refuse sex (Panel Study)

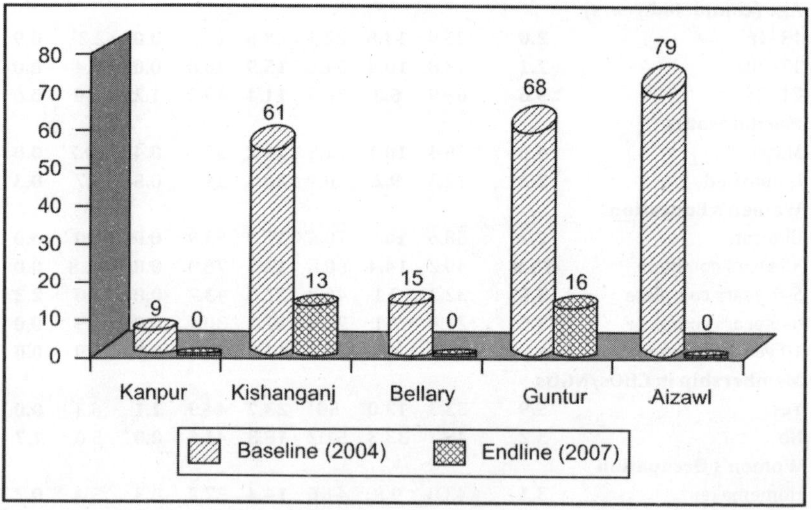

However, despite the overall decrease in the reporting of inability by women to refuse sex, insights from views and opinions of local key informants and focus group discussions highlight inherent vulnerabilities of women and to exert sexual rights in a society deep rooted in culture and tradition.

Poverty, low social status and lack of equal economic rights and opportunities make girls and women susceptible to sexual trafficking and exploitation and exchanging sexual favours for necessities and goods. Sheer IEC awareness programmes and discussions of women rights will not reduce the vulnerability of women and reduce the gap in empowering them. Therefore, addressing gender roles and power dynamics between women and men, and how they impact on sexual relations and decision-making is critical for effective prevention. Sustained programmes according to the needs and tailored responses that foster gender equality are critical for success: while girls and women must be empowered, boys and men should be enabled to become supportive, responsible partners in internalizing the positive perception or attitudinal changes in the lives of women.

Perception related to sexual rights

Table 4.7 presents the data pertaining to the perception of young women that a husband should be accepted under any condition even if he has extra-marital relationship. The survey shows that the perception varies very strikingly. As seen in Table 4.7, a smaller proportion of unmarried young women across all the states aged 13–16 perceive that the husband should be accepted if he has extra-marital relations. However, it is noteworthy that a larger majority of women aged 17–20 in Kishanganj (9%), Bellary (44%) and those aged 21–24 in Kanpur (9%) and Guntur (9%) believe that the husband should be accepted despite his extra-marital relations. The only exception is in Aizawl, where the response remains similar across all age groups in baseline findings and none (zero representation) in the endline findings across all background characteristics. It reflects that women in Aizawl are not ready to accept the husband's extra-marital relations. Interestingly, except in Aizawl, across all the study areas more married women are of the opinion that a husband should be accepted under any condition compared to the unmarried young women. This finding in a way reflects the Indian tradition of maintaining the marriage and acceptance of husband's behaviours.

Education also has a positive impact on young women's perception that husband should be accepted under any condition, even if he has extra-marital relations. Higher acceptance of husband's extra-marital relations is reported by illiterate women in Kanpur (13%), Bellary (45%) and Guntur (8%). However, in Kishanganj, more literate women accepted husband's extra-marital relations (9%) compared to illiterate women (7%). Such a perception also reflects the strong cultural/traditional influences and low status accorded to women despite their education. Women in salaried/paid jobs also show more acceptances of husband's extra-marital relations compared to homemakers and those working as labourers or in family farms.

Exposure to mass media has a positive impact in acceptance of husband's extra-marital relations. In Kanpur, Bellary and Guntur women who are exposed to media reported lower acceptance of

Table 4.7

Percentage of young women who perceived husband should be accepted under any condition even he has extra-marital relationship by selected characteristics and districts

Background characteristics	*Kanpur**	*Kishanganj*		*Bellary*		*Guntur*		*Aizawl*	
	EL	*BL*	*EL*	*BL*	*EL*	*BL*	*EL*	*BL*	*EL*
Age (completed years)									
13–16	**4.5**	6.3	**4.6**	35	**34.1**	9.2	**3.1**	6.6	**0.0**
17–20	**5.7**	18.2	**9.2**	59.4	**44.0**	9.0	**4.5**	6.9	**0.0**
21–24	**9.2**	25.6	**8.9**	56.8	**42.0**	15.7	**6.1**	6.9	**0.0**
Marital Status									
Married	**9.0**	29.7	**11.7**	63.4	**48.3**	12.9	**6.4**	4.8	**0.0**
Unmarried	**5.0**	6.2	**3.7**	35.6	**33.0**	8.5	**2.7**	7.2	**0.0**
Women's Education									
Illiterate	**13.0**	23.9	**7.1**	70.8	**45.2**	17.1	**7.7**	0.0	**0.0**
<5 years complete	**15.0**	12.5	**9.1**	53.8	**46.7**	20.0	**9.1**	0.0	**0.0**
5–7 years complete	**8.5**	12.6	**11.5**	54.1	**37.8**	13.0	**5.6**	8.0	**0.0**
8–9 years complete	**5.6**	7.3	**5.4**	34.2	**40.2**	6.7	**1.6**	6.1	**0.0**
10 and above	**4.0**	10.2	**6.6**	23.5	**32.6**	3.9	**2.9**	7.5	**0.0**
Membership in CBOs/NGOs									
Yes	**5.9**	16.7	**8.7**	54.5	**36.1**	16.7	**6.1**	4.5	**0.0**
No	**4.8**	16.2	**0.0**	51.7	**44.7**	9.9	**3.8**	9.9	**0.0**
Women's Occupation									
Homemaker	**6.1**	14.8	**8.0**	41.8	**34.2**	33.3	**5.4**	7.1	**0.0**
Working as labourer/family farm	**12.5**	47.4	0.0	69.2	**48.4**	8.4	**1.2**	7.3	**0.0**
Salaried/paid job	**0.0**	0.0	**20.0**	50.0	**51.6**	14.8	**25**	0.0	**0.0**
Migratory Status of Husband									
Non-migrant	**10.0**	15.1	**9.2**	51.6	**47.4**	10.7	**6.2**	6.8	**0.0**
Migrant	**7.1**	38.5	**18.6**	100.0	**50.0**	50.0	**7.1**	0.0	**0.0**
Exposure to Mass Media									
Yes	**5.7**	13.9	**9.0**	48.4	**38.8**	9.8	**4.7**	6.8	**0.0**
No	**11.1**	24.2	**5.2**	83.3	**51.8**	16.2	**7.7**	0.0	**0.0**
Total (N)	**6.3**	16.1	**8.0**	51.6	**40.1**	10.6	**4.8**	6.8	**0**
	(494)	(539)	**(465)**	(488)	**(556)**	(472)	**(417)**	(471)	**(439)**

* Information from the baseline survey is not presented due to change in intervention after the baseline survey.

husband's extra-marital relations compared to those who are not exposed to media (11% in Kanpur, 52% in Bellary and 8% in Guntur). However, in Kishanganj, it shows a reverse pattern: an increase in acceptance of husband's extra-marital relations with exposure to media. Compared with non-migrants, those women having migrant husbands perceive that the husband's extra-marital relations should be accepted. In Kishanganj, Bellary and Guntur, women whose husbands have migrated to other places are ready to accept their husband's extra-marital relations. This figure is higher in Bellary than in the other districts.

Looking at the overall data and comparing with the baseline findings, there are changes in accepting husband's extra-marital relations under any condition. There is a drastic reduction and the proportion goes down from 31 per cent to 6 per cent in Kanpur, 16 per cent to 8 per cent in Kishanganj, 52 per cent to 40 per cent in Bellary, 11 per cent to 5 per cent in Guntur and 7 per cent to zero per cent in Aizawl.

Sexual violence

The charter on reproductive and sexual rights of women entails that a woman has the right to be free from torture and ill-treatment and can be used for campaigning for protection from rape, sexual assault and sexual abuse, coercion to engage in any unlawful sexual activities, sexual harassment and violence including domestic violence. Despite these rights, there is a severe threat to women's autonomy in safe sexual negotiations. A considerable proportion of women in almost every socio-economic set-up are still ill-treated and the magnitude of sexual violence which includes forced/coerced sex or rape has definitely a detrimental effect on woman's physical and mental health. Such violence also leaves a woman at high risk of acquiring STIs and HIV due to her subordinate position.

Table 4.8 presents reports of sexual violence by young women over the period. Baseline survey results of Kishanganj show 41 per cent women had experienced forced penetrative sex, while in Bellary it was 38 per cent and relatively low in the other districts. The proportion varies from 3 per cent in Aizawl to 17 per cent in Guntur. Nearly half the women in Bellary (46%) reported that their husbands do not respect their decisions about unwillingness to have sex. The figure for the other districts is relatively low and it varies between 2 per cent in Aizawl and 24 per cent in Kishanganj. The endline survey shows a decrease in women reporting forced penetrative sex with 26 per cent in Kishanganj, 25 per cent in Bellary and 1 per cent in Aizawl.

There is an increase in women reporting forced penetrative sex in Guntur (22.5%). There has been a decrease in reporting of husband does not respect their decision about unwillingness to have sex from 46 per cent to 23 per cent in Bellary, and in Aizawl it decreases from 2 per cent to 1 per cent. In the other districts there is an increase in this case, varying from five per cent to 18 per cent in Guntur, 24 per cent to 25 per cent in Kishanganj.

Table 4.8

Percentage of women reporting sexual violence in the five CHARCA districts

(%)

Sexual violence and coercion	*Kanpur**	*Kishanganj*		*Bellary*		*Guntur*		*Aizawl*	
	EL (494)	*BL (539)*	*EL (865)*	*BL (488)*	*EL (556)*	*BL (472)*	*EL (417)*	*BL (471)*	*EL (439)*
Women reporting forced penetrative sex	**24.7**	41.4	**26.0**	38.3	**24.5**	16.7	**22.5**	2.8	**1.1***
Women whose husbands do not respect their decision about their unwillingness for sex	**20.2**	23.9	**25.4**	45.9	**22.7**	4.9	**17.7**	2.1	**1.4***

* Information from the baseline survey is not presented due to change in intervention after the baseline survey.

Table 4.9

Extent of sexual coercion/violence reported by young men in the five CHARCA districts (%)

Sexual violence and coercion	*Kanpur**	*Kishanganj*		*Bellary*		*Guntur*		*Aizawl*	
	EL	*BL*	*EL*	*BL*	*EL*	*BL*	*EL*	*BL*	*EL*
Young men who often have sex with their partner if they are unwilling	**32.9**	34.7	**8.8**	6.3	**30**	34.5	**19.6**	15.9	**3.3**
Young men who do not respect women decision if she don't want sex	**28.3**	32.3	**12.5**	3.1	**34.7**	21.6	**13.6**	21.6	**2.2**
Total	**322**	291	**328**	256	**317**	264	**214**	220	**184**

* Information from the baseline survey is not presented due to change in intervention after the baseline survey.

Table 4.9 shows the extent of sexual violence/coercion reported by young men in the baseline and endline surveys. The baseline data reveals that in Kishanganj 32 per cent of the males reported that they do not respect a woman's decision if she does not want sex. However, it is quite encouraging to note that around 90 per cent of the males in Kanpur, Guntur and Aizawl respect their wife's decision if she does not want sex. Male behaviour regarding sexual violence is quite favourable for women except in Kishanganj and Guntur. In the endline survey,

> '... the situation regarding women's life has changed lot in this community ... earlier there were lots of cases where a single woman going for fetching water or for some other reason on the outskirts the village gets abused by boys ... but now people have changed ... women are feeling safe to go out even alone and doing outside household activities like shopping and visiting friends in nearby village ...'
>
> —Man, FGD, Kishanganj
>
> '... now girls in our village are bold enough to react ... they don't keep silent on any misbehaviour by anyone inside or outside the home. They go to school with boys, competing on many occasions with boys ... even many times boys also seek our help in studies and other things ... we have found the boys have a respect for girls ... they behave nicely while dealing with us ...'
>
> —Woman KI, Guntur
>
> '... behaving with an intention to dominate the women at every field is not a human quality ... if we think that man is powerful then ideally power is to protect not to abuse ... earlier few cases were found like wife beating and other mistreatment against women in our villages but now there is no such mishappening for past few years ...'
>
> —Man KI, Aizawl
>
> '... many times we blame others for abusing the women at different levels. But it is also true that violence happens within family too. In this community, I know some cases of domestic abuse ... I have talked to women whose husbands often force them to have sex even if they are not well or not ready for ...'
>
> —Peer educator, FGD, Bellary
>
> '... Men never consider women as human beings ... teasing the young girls is often seen in the community ... girls coming from tuition classes in late evening feel scared of boys in the market. In some cases boys do many filthy things with women standing in the overcrowded bus ...'
>
> —Woman KI, Kanpur

reporting of forced sex increased from 6 per cent to 30 per cent in Bellary. In other districts, a decrease in reporting of forced/coerced sex is observed with the lowest of 3 per cent in Aizawl. Kishanganj shows a drastic improvement in decreasing the vulnerability of women. The reported figures of men having forced sex with their partners against their willingness vary strikingly across the states, with a high of 33 per cent in Kanpur to a low of 3 per cent in Aizawl. As in the baseline findings, it is encouraging to observe that a considerable proportion of men in Kanpur (72%), Kishanganj (88%), Guntur (86%) and Aizawl (98%) respect their wife's decision if she does not want sex. In Bellary 35 per cent do not respect women's such decision. Comparison of data shows that in Bellary the number of men who do not respect women's decision increased from three per cent in the baseline survey to 35 per cent in the endline survey.

Sexual and power dynamics have always marginalized the womenfolk across the culture. The traditional norms and practices, particularly in a cultural set-up like India, where the man has always enjoyed a better power authority than the woman, have been a challenge for all intervening factors. Affecting the strong rooted sexual power of men across the five districts uniformly is certainly a difficult task for the CHARCA programmes. That is what exactly the qualitative findings bring out while exploring this issue. There is a district-wise variation in improving the women's experience and men's reorganization of women sexual rights which lies at par with the survey findings too. However, it is a welcoming scenario that the women's sexual rights and perspectives have improved in three districts. The evident fact of synergizing men's sensitization of sustainable realization of women's sexual rights has been seen while exploring the issue of women sexual rights from men and women both across the five CHARCA districts.

Condom use during the last sexual encounter

In the context of HIV/AIDS, where young men and women are particularly at a higher risk of getting infected, correct and consistent use of condom, apart from sexual abstinence, serves as a protection not only against unwanted pregnancy but also against HIV and other sexually transmitted infections (STIs). However, with reference to condom as a method of contraception and protection against STIs/HIV, although young women's and men's knowledge of condom use may be relatively good, literature suggests that condom may not be popularly used as there is much of male resistance to its use, unequal power relations/dynamics, negative attitude attached to it and that it may also be unlikely to be used in a stable, ongoing relationship or whose family size is not complete.

In this backdrop, it is of interest to know whether young women used condom during the last sexual encounter, and if they are aware about condom protecting them from STIs. This indirectly helps us in knowing the status of women and their sexual rights in negotiating safer sex.

Table 4.10

Percentage of women reporting use of condom during last sexual encounter

Use of condoms	*Kanpur**	*Kishanganj*		*Bellary*		*Guntur*		*Aizawl*	
	EL	*BL*	*EL*	*BL*	*EL*	*BL*	*EL*	*BL*	*EL*
Young women reporting use of condom during last sexual encounter	13.2	25.0	17.4	1.1	5.6	2.0	7.6	7.8	8.9
Total	(175)	(539)	(258)	(488)	(268)	(472)	(236)	(471)	(75)

* Information from the baseline survey is not presented due to change in intervention after the baseline survey.

Figure 4.2

Proportion of young women using condom in the last encounter (Panel Study)

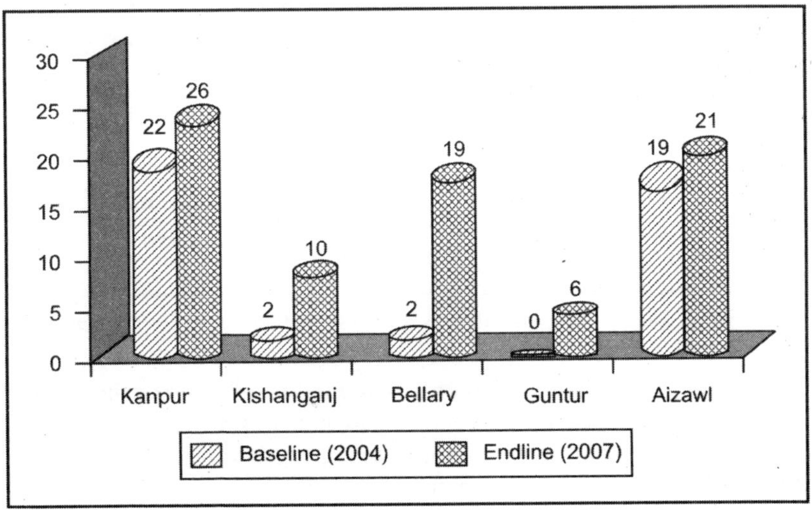

Table 4.10 presents condom use in the last sexual encounter reported by young women. Except for Kishanganj, young women reporting use of condom during the last sexual encounter increased from 1 per cent to 6 per cent in Bellary, 2 per cent to 8 per cent in Guntur and 8 to 9 per cent in Aizawl. The increase in reporting condom use during the last sexual encounter to a certain extent highlights the increase in women's awareness about sexual and reproductive health. It also shows the negotiating power of women for safer sex with their partners. In Kishanganj, however, young women reporting use of condom during the last sexual encounter decreased from 25 to 17 per cent.

The panel data, as presented in Figure 4.2, show increased improvement in condom use during last sexual encounter (despite its low use) in all the CHARCA districts. The increase reflects the efficacy of programme implementation, which shows an increase by 8 per cent in Guntur (2 to 10%), 17 per cent in Aizawl (2 to 19%), 6 per cent in Bellary (0 to 6%) and 2 per cent in Kishanganj (19 to 21%). Overall, Aizawl district shows the highest increase in the proportion of young women using condom during the last sexual encounter.

Table 4.11

Percentage of women reporting condom use during last sexual encounter by their awareness about location and correct use of condom

		*Kanpur**	*Kishanganj*		*Bellary*		*Guntur*		*Aizawl*	
		EL	*BL*	*EL*	*BL*	*EL*	*BL*	*EL*	*BL*	*EL*
Locations to get a male condom	Knows no source	**18.2**	6.0	**0.0**	0.8	**1.1**	0.0	**3.1**	7.9	**0.0**
	Knows at least one source	**43.5**	34.1	**34.1**	3.1	**8.0**	8.1	**8.3**	8.2	**52.0**
Correct use of condom can prevent STI infection	Yes	**43.8**	29.2	**23.8**	8.3	**9.5**	8.3	**8.2**	5.5	**52.0**
	No	**0.0**	26.3	**8.2**	0.0	**0.0**	0.0	**0.0**	25.0	**0.0**

* Information from the baseline survey is not presented due to change in intervention after the baseline survey.

Table 4.11 shows women's knowledge about the source of getting condom and its correct use in prevention of STI infection among women who used condom during the last sexual encounter. Despite reporting condom use during the last sexual encounter, there are still sections of women who do not know any source of getting male condom. It ranges from 1 per cent in Bellary to 18 per cent in Kanpur in the endline study. Knowing at least one source of getting male condom among those who used it during the last sexual encounter varies from a high of 52 per cent in Aizawl to a low of 8 per cent in Bellary. Comparison between the baseline and endline surveys shows an increase in the awareness/knowledge of women in getting male condom.

It is encouraging to observe in the endline study that among those women who used condom during the last sexual encounter, there were no women who did not know that the correct and consistent use of condom can prevent them from STIs. More than half the women in Aizawl (52%) and 44 per cent in Kanpur who used condom during the last sexual encounter knew that the correct use of condom can prevent them from STIs. The corresponding figures for other districts range from 8 per cent in Guntur to 24 per cent in Kishanganj.

The finding is, to an extent, encouraging though condom use is still low across all the districts. Overall, there is an improvement in the use of condom, suggesting gaining acceptance of condom by young women. This finding is encouraging, given the increase in the use of condom both in cross-sectional study (three CHARCA districts) and panel study (across all CHARCA districts) but it remains incomplete with a mere assessment of condom use during the last sexual encounter without understanding the reasons for condom use, the context in which they use and the women who use condoms. Awareness/knowledge of condoms is obviously a necessary, if not sufficient, condition for their acceptance and use. But beliefs about condom, both positive and negative, are also likely to influence its use. It is therefore necessary to find the possible explanations about the motivations or barriers to use condom. There is clearly a need to ascertain the methods young men and women use to protect themselves against risks. Understanding the factors that influence condom use could improve interventions that are aimed at encouraging protective behaviour to reduce the dual risks of unwanted pregnancy and HIV infection. The study's findings may have limited generalizations, as interpretation of the findings is limited by the focus on condom use during the last sexual intercourse. It suggests that given the role of condom in protecting against both risks – pregnancy/ STI/HIV infections, providers should address them as interrelated. Specifically, providers should focus their counseling on correct and consistent use of condom in combination with the use of other contraceptives. Directly addressing the dual risks of pregnancy and HIV infection would dramatically improve the level of condom use.

Summary of findings and conclusions

- Impact of CHARCA intervention in enhancing awareness among women of their reproductive rights has not emerged significantly. There has been a significant decline in the proportion of women, who feel that they are free to exercise their reproductive rights. In fact, these are the cultural issues rooted in the process of socialization and hence any programme for such a short duration may not impact the value system. This is why, even when a considerable proportion of women are aware of these issues, it is not reflected in their perception and behaviour. However, this proportion has increased in the case of panel data.
- Across all the districts, less than one in five young women does not have the ability to refuse sex, and this inability increases in younger age group, low literacy, non-members of CBOs/NGOs. However, there is significant increase in the proportion of women who have the ability to refuse sex.
- Except in Aizawl, all the districts indicate substantial increase in the proportion of women who are agreed that husbands should be accepted despite extra-marital relations. This proportion is high in case of married and older women.
- The proportion of women who reported forced penetrative sex declined significantly between the two rounds of CHARCA surveys, lowest in Aizawl and highest in Bellary. Similarly, a decrease is observed in reporting that husbands do not respect their decisions about unwillingness to have sex.
- There has been a substantial decrease in the incidence of forced sex in Aizawl, Kishanganj and Guntur. Likewise, in Kanpur, Guntur and Aizawl more men reported in the endline survey that they respect their wife's decision if they do not want sex. This is a significant improvement over the baseline survey.
- Condom use during the last sexual encounter declined in three districts. However, panel data reflects a significant improvement in condom use during the last sexual encounter.

5

Violence Against Women and Support System

Violence against women or domestic violence in any form (physical, psychological or sexual) generates wide interest in population and health studies due to its direct link with their status as well as vulnerability in the society. Around the world, on an average, one in every three women is mistreated, beaten or coerced into sex, or otherwise abused in her lifetime (Kishor and Johnson, 2004). Studies indicate growing evidence of an increase in violence against women across different boundaries of culture, cutting across age, class, education, income and ethnicity for various reasons (Goode, 1971; Dyson and Moore, 1982; Rao, 1998; Bloch and Rao, 2002; Eswaran and Malhotra; IIPS and Macro International, 2007). Women and girls are the frequent victims of physical violence within the family and between intimate partners accompanied by severe psychological and verbal abuse.

The other interest in domestic violence is its association with reproductive health beyond pregnancy and childbearing outcomes, such as their vulnerability to the risk of HIV and sexually transmitted infections (STIs), reproductive decision-making and contraceptive use. Specially pernicious is that violence has a significant impact on women's health responsible for one in every five potential years of healthy life lost (WHO and UNAIDS, 2000).

The CHARCA project, in view of enabling young women towards increased knowledge and protection from HIV/AIDS, also aims to empower women in terms of their rights and ability to protect themselves from physical and sexual abuse through improved community level support and leadership. In this context, the present chapter explains violence against women and the support system experienced by young women in the project areas through

- issues discussed in CBOs/NGOs,
- awareness and capacity building by CBOs/NGOs,
- violence against women, and
- support system for women.

Functioning of CBOs/NGOs

Issues discussed at meetings

The functioning of CBO/NGOs is important in a community, especially in a rural set-up, in view of their potentially significant contributions towards awareness and enhancement of people's rights and responsibilities and overall development of the society. The role of NGOs and other developmental programmes in diffusing awareness is largely recognized across the districts uniformly which got reflected in the qualitative findings. Similar to the baseline survey, in the endline survey also, the young women (aged 13–25 years) were asked about the functioning of CBOs/NGOs in and around their community and issues addressed by such organizations.

Table 5.1

Percentage of women reporting issues discussed in CBO/NGO meetings during the last 12 months in the five CHARCA districts

Issues discussed	*Kanpur**	*Kishanganj*		*Bellary*		*Guntur*		*Aizawl*	
	EL (494)	*BL (539)*	*EL (465)*	*BL (488)*	*EL (556)*	*BL (472)*	*EL (417)*	*BL (471)*	*EL (439)*
Membership in CBOs/NGOs	**3.4**	1.1	**4.9**	4.5	**17.4**	4.6	**42.2**	57.1	**86.6**
Women's rights	**64.2**	65.4	**66.7**	13.1	**83.3**	10.3	**71.3**	43.8	**94.5**
STI/RTI/HIV	**73.4**	46.2	**45.8**	5.0	**84.5**	5.2	**91.0**	76.2	**99.7**
Violence against young women	**62.1**	30.8	**58.3**	8.8	**68.6**	7.9	**22.8**	38.6	**93.8**
Total Women	**(271)**	(26)	**(24)**	(160)	**(354)**	(253)	**(400)**	(260)	**(985)**

* Information from the baseline survey is not presented due to change in intervention after the baseline survey.

Note: BL = baseline survey in 2004 and EL= endline survey in 2007.

As shown in Table 5.1 and Figure 5.1, the number of women having membership in CBOs/NGOs in the endline survey is highest in Aizawl (87%), followed by Guntur (42%), Bellary (17%), Kishanganj (5%) and least in Kanpur (3%). Further, the data reveals that in Aizawl, Kanpur, Bellary and Guntur, issues of STI/RTI/HIV have been mostly discussed, followed by women's rights and violence against women. However, in Kishanganj rights of women (67%) was the major issue discussed in the CBO/NGO meetings, followed by violence (58%), and 46 per cent women reported discussions about of STI/RTI/HIV.

Figure 5.1

Membership of women in CBOs/NGOs

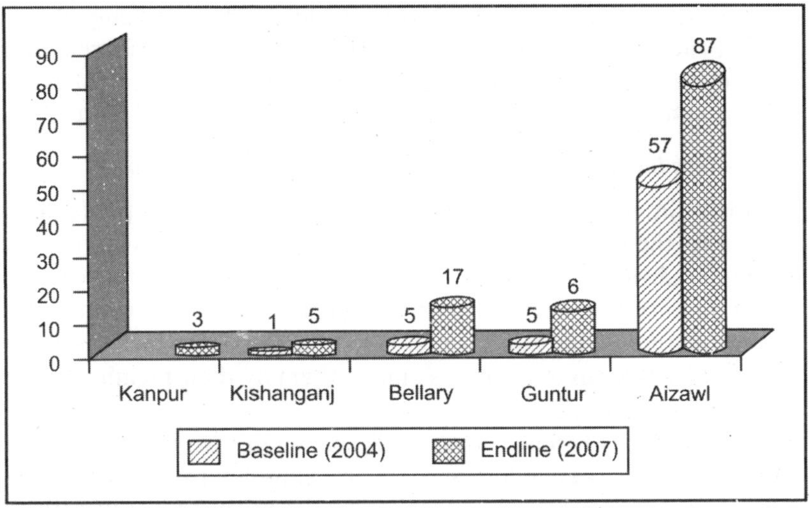

Issues pertaining STI/RTI/HIV were mainly discussed in the CBO/NGO meetings in Aizawl (100%), followed by 91 per cent in Guntur, 85 per cent in Bellary and 73 per cent in Kanpur. These were, however, less discussed in Kishanganj (46%). In the case of discussing women's rights in meetings, 95 per cent women in Aizawl, 83 per cent in Bellary 71 per cent in Guntur, 67 per cent in Kishanganj and 64 per cent in Kanpur reported the discussion. The issue of violence was discussed mostly in Aizawl (94%), and to some extent in Bellary (69%), Kanpur (62%) and Kishanganj (58%), while only 23 per cent of women reported it being discussed in Guntur.

Overall, a considerable improvement is indicated over the baseline survey, on various issues discussed in the meetings of CBOs/NGOs. About 80–86 per cent increase is noted in reporting

> '... the NGO working in this area provides a congenial environment for us to gain information on HIV/AIDS prevention, sexual health problems, family planning, self-help groups, health and nutritional care for infants and ways to open up and feel free with family members and freely exercise personal rights ...'
>
> —Female KI, Kanpur

discussion of STI/RTI/HIV issues in the districts of Bellary and Guntur and a 65 per cent increase in Kanpur. However, there has been a slight decrease reported in Kishanganj. A 70 per cent and 60 per cent increase is seen in the case of women's rights in Bellary and Guntur respectively and a marginal increase is indicated in Kishanganj. The issue of violence discussed in CBO/NGO meetings has also increased in the endline survey by 60 per cent in Bellary, 55 per cent in Aizawl and to some extent (about 15–28%) in Guntur, Kishanganj and Kanpur.

Awareness level among women by CBO/NGO membership

The CHARCA endline survey attempts to assess women's perceptions related to their reproductive health, focusing on the awareness of women regarding the availability of male condom and its preventive utility against STIs/HIV as well as the importance of maintaining sexual relations with one partner. Women have also been assessed about HIV/AIDS misconceptions among them by their membership in community organizations.

Table 5.2 presents awareness of young women regarding knowledge of use of condom and HIV transmission by membership in CBOs/NGOs. In general, more women who are members of CBOs/NGOs reported having knowledge of at least one location of getting male condom and also its role in prevention of HIV in all the districts except in Kishanganj. On the contrary, women who are not members are better aware of the importance of having sex with one partner to curb HIV in the districts of Kishanganj, Guntur and Bellary. In Kishanganj and Bellary having one misconception of HIV/AIDS transmission is higher among women who are members of CBOs/NGOs.

Among women having membership in CBOs/NGOs, the knowledge about at least one location of getting male condom, its protective function against HIV as well as knowing that sex with one partner can protect a person from STIs/HIV is highest in Kanpur and Aizawl and lowest in Kishanganj. Misconceptions regarding

HIV/AIDS transmission among women are more prevalent in Bellary and Kishanganj compared to Aizawl, irrespective of CBO/NGO membership.

Table 5.2

Awareness among young women regarding knowledge of source and use of condom and misconception of HIV transmission by membership in CBOs/NGOs (%)

District	*Survey*	*Membership of CBOs/ NGOs*	*At least one location of male condom is known*	*Knowing that consistent use of condom can protect a person from STIs/HIV*	*Knowing that sex with one partner can protect a person from acquiring STIs/HIV*	*Having one misconception of HIV/AIDS transmission is known*
Kanpur*	**EL**	**Yes**	**100.0**	**100.0**	**100.0**	**11.8**
		No	**69.5**	**92.4**	**82.3**	**14.6**
Kishanganj	BL	Yes	66.7	83.3	100	100
		No	55.5	58.3	40.2	62.3
	EL	**Yes**	**47.8**	**63.2**	**57.9**	**47.8**
		No	**66.7**	**100.0**	**100.0**	**33.3**
Bellary	BL	Yes	22.7	45.5	81.8	86.4
		No	11.2	23.4	68.7	71
	EL	**Yes**	**85.6**	**95.5**	**84.8**	**79.4**
		No	**83.3**	**95.1**	**85.9**	**74.7**
Guntur	BL	Yes	31.9	23.2	55.1	72.5
		No	18.6	27.3	51.2	67.2
	EL	**Yes**	**83.0**	**98.1**	**98.1**	**10.2**
		No	**85.0**	**97.5**	**98.5**	**12.3**
Aizawl	BL	Yes	50.9	92.6	89.2	93.3
		No	29.7	87.1	78.7	92.1
	EL	**Yes**	**91.9**	**100.0**	**100.0**	**3.9**
		No	**84.5**	**100.0**	**100.0**	**17.2**

* Information from the baseline survey is not presented due to change in intervention after the baseline survey.

All women in Kanpur, who are members of CBOs/NGOs, know all the three different types of knowledge issues asked, while in Aizawl it is with knowledge related to consistent use of condom and sex with one partner as a means of HIV prevention. It is also observed that across all districts, a gap exists between the knowledge of condom use to prevent HIV/AIDS and the knowledge of at least one location to get male condom, suggesting the need to improve availability of condoms as well as awareness about their locations. The gap is highest in Kishanganj, followed by Kanpur, Aizawl, Bellary and Guntur.

A comparison of baseline and endline surveys indicates that among women with membership in CBOs/NGOs, the knowledge of at least one location of male condom has increased by 40 to 60 per cent in the districts of Bellary, Guntur and Aizawl and the knowledge of use of condom as a means of HIV prevention increased by 50 per cent in Bellary and 70 per cent in Guntur. Knowledge of having sex with one partner to curb the spread of HIV has risen by 40 per cent each in Kishanganj and Guntur. Kishanganj shows a decline of 20 to 40 per cent in the three types of knowledge among women who are members of CBOs/NGOs. Also, there has been a decline in the proportion of women having at least one misconception about HIV/AIDS transmission in all the districts. Similarly, there has been a 90 per cent decline in the number of women having one HIV/AIDS misconception in Kanpur and Aizawl, while a 60 per cent and 50 per cent decline is reported in Guntur and Kishanganj respectively.

Capacity building by CBO/NGO membership

The survey also assessed the gap between perceived sexual rights and the behavioural aspect of sexual rights among young women aged 13–24 years about acceptance of husband's extra-marital relations and their ability to refuse conjugal sex.

Table 5.3 presents women's perceptions of sexual rights by membership in CBOs/NGOs, which shows not much difference between women who are members and those who are not in terms of their sexual rights. Only in Bellary, none of women having membership in CBOs/NGOs reported that they do not accept husband's extra-marital relations. In the case of not having ability to refuse sex if she is not willing, the proportion is lower among those having membership in CBOs/NGOs, except in Bellary.

The proportions of young women perceiving that husbands should be accepted even after their extra-marital affairs as well as those who do not have the ability to refuse sex when not willing are highest in Bellary than other districts. The survey results clearly bring out the importance of membership of CBOs/NGOs in empowering women about their sexual rights.

Considering the improvement in endline over the baseline survey, it can be inferred that overall there has been an increase in the sexual rights of women in all the districts. In terms of women perceiving acceptance of husbands even after their extra-marital relations, a decline of 34 per cent in Kanpur, 15 per cent in Bellary and ten per cent in Guntur has been marked. With respect to behaviour regarding sexual rights, the proportion of women who lack ability to refuse sex has also decreased by 53 per cent in Kishanganj, 30 per cent in Bellary, seven per cent in Guntur. However, this proportion has slightly risen by six per cent in Kanpur.

Table 5.3

Percentage of women about their sexual rights by membership in CBOs/NGOs

District	*Survey*	*Membership in CBOs/NGOs*	*Young women perceive that a husband should be accepted under any condition even he has extra-marital relations*	*Young women who don't have ability to refuse sex if they are not willing*
Kanpur*	**EL**	**Yes**	**5.9**	**5.9**
		No	**4.8**	**3.2**
Kishanganj	BL	Yes	16.9	66.7
		No	16.2	36.2
	EL	**Yes**	**0.0**	**13.0**
		No	**0.0**	**33.3**
Bellary	BL	Yes	54.5	64.2
		No	51.7	48.5
	EL	**Yes**	**36.1**	**23.7**
		No	**44.7**	**18.3**
Guntur	BL	Yes	16.7	8.5
		No	9.9	5.9
	EL	**Yes**	**5.7**	**1.1**
		No	**3.8**	**0.0**
Aizawl	BL	Yes	4.5	8.7
		No	9.9	2.5
	EL	**Yes**	**0.0**	**0.0**
		No	**0.0**	**1.7**

* Information from the baseline survey is not presented due to change in intervention after the baseline survey.

Women's autonomy and role in decision-making

Participation of women in decision-making on issues related to health and activities in community is important for the betterment of women's status and their empowerment. To comprehend the extent of empowerment among women in terms of decision-making, young women aged 13–24 were asked about their perception of needing permission from their husbands on some issues.

Table 5.4 and Figures 5.2a and 5.2b present the responses of women related to their mobility aspects across the CHARCA districts. In Kanpur women mostly do not need permission from their husbands to visit the neighbourhood (10%) but most of them require permission to visit their natal family. In Kishanganj, 25 per cent women do not need permission from their husbands to participate in the CBO/NGO meetings but most women require permission to visit the neighbourhood. Similarly, in Bellary, women are also fairly empowered to attend CBO/NGO meetings (17%) but they have least freedom in visiting health services. In Guntur and Aizawl most women do not need permission to visit the neighbourhood, but women in Guntur are least empowered to participate in CBO/NGO meetings. In Aizawl least freedom exists among women in visiting their natal family.

Table 5.4

Percentage of married women who never seek husband's permission on mobility aspects

Mobility parameters	*Kanpur**	*Kishanganj*		*Bellary*		*Guntur*		*Aizawl*	
	EL	*BL*	*EL*	*BL*	*EL*	*BL*	*EL*	*BL*	*EL*
Visiting health services	**3.6**	7.3	**17.7**	2.5	**0.8**	10	**1.7**	4.9	**0.0**
Visiting natal family	**1.2**	0.9	**14.9**	4.2	**16.5**	10.3	**3.0**	20.7	**4.2**
Visiting neighbourhood	**9.5**	7.3	**8.5**	33.5	**1.9**	31.3	**42.6**	19.8	**8.3**
Participating in CBO/NGO meetings	**8.3**	76.5	**25.4**	0.4	**17.2**	22.3	**1.3**	18.8	**6.9**
Total Women	**169**	234	**248**	284	**261**	252	**235**	82	**72**

* Information from the baseline survey is not presented due to change in intervention after the baseline survey.

Figure 5.2a

Women not needing permission for utilization of health services (%)

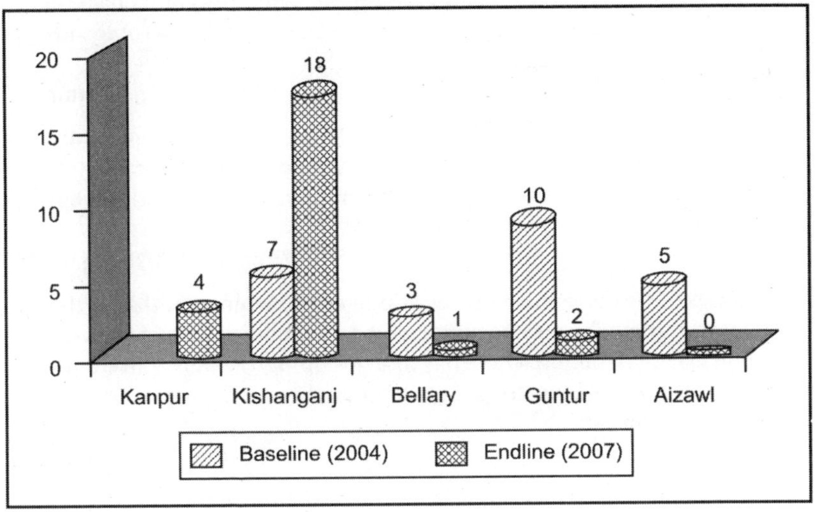

Figure 5.2b

Women not needing permission to participate in CBOs/NGOs (%)

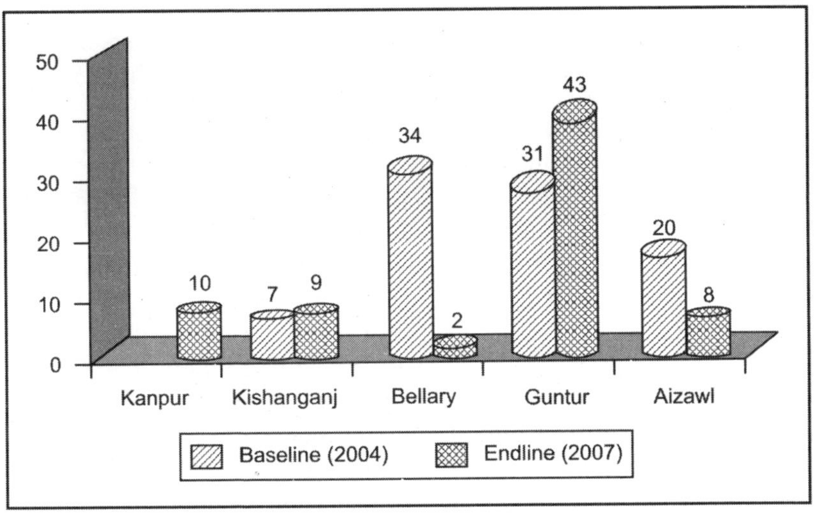

> '... I and my daughter went to attend a meeting where information regarding HIV/AIDS and family planning was being provided when my husband also arrived. He became furious and brought us back to home and scolded me that their daughter can choose the wrong path after hearing those things ...'
>
> —Woman KI, Kanpur
>
> '... women in our community have to take permission in each and every matter of life ... doing without the approval of husband is not considered a good behaviour in our community. It's the practice what we can do ...'
>
> —Woman KI, Kishanganj
>
> '... men used to show their ownership over the women ... that is the reason why they always check the women's mobility ... husbands do nothing except drinking whole day and gossiping ... when wife comes home from work she has to give explanation before husband why she is late by few minutes ...'
>
> —Peer educator, FGD, Bellary
>
> '... my husband used to ask some time where I am going and why I am going ... now when he saw I am earning more than him, he never says anything to me. Now I take most of the decisions in our family ... even sometimes for my husband ...'
>
> —Woman KI, Guntur
>
> '... women can go to market, to visit friends and have some break with peers ... they don't ask for permission if it is for short time ... for longer period visits you need to discuss with your husband or other family members not because of allowing but for other logistics of managing home and family ...'
>
> —Woman FGD, Aizawl

Regarding visiting health centres, more women in Kishanganj (18%) are empowered to take independent decisions in comparison to the other districts. But the proportion of women requiring permission to visit their natal family is highest in Bellary (17%), followed by 15 per cent in Kishanganj, and in the remaining districts the proportion is negligible. Similarly regarding permission needed to visit the neighbourhood, over two-fifths of the women in Guntur (43%) do not need husband's permission while in the rest of the districts more women seek permission from households. In Kishanganj one-fifth of the women and 17 per cent in Bellary are empowered to participate in the meetings of CBOs/NGOs compared to 7 to 8 per cent in Aizawl and Kanpur and 1 per cent in Guntur.

Looking at the changes in the endline survey results over the baseline survey findings, it can be observed that except for a 10 per cent increase in Kishanganj, there has been a decline of 12 per cent in Kanpur, 8 per cent in Guntur and 2 per cent in Bellary in the proportion of women not requiring permission from their husbands to visit health services. Similarly, there has been a decrease in the number of women not needing permission to visit their natal family in all the districts, especially Aizawl (17%), except in Kishanganj which has shown an increase of 14 per cent. The proportion of women having freedom to participate in CBO/NGO meetings has also shown a decline – 51 per cent in Kishanganj, 28 per cent in Kanpur and 21 per cent in Guntur. Nevertheless, Bellary and Aizawl have shown an increase of 21 per cent and 12 per cent respectively in this case.

The independence of women and their activities are still under men's dominance and approval. Qualitative findings reveal many instances of male intervention in women's activities such as mobility. In many cases the women's vulnerability is getting reflected.

Violence against women

Studies indicate that domestic violence is pervasive and reflects power relationship and social control over women. Violence meted out to women ranges from casual, individual, non-formal acts to more planned, organized and systematic ones. Domestic violence may take the forms of physical, sexual, verbal, social, emotional, financial, intellectual violence, state, communal or caste instigated violence while some others may include not letting women to avail educational opportunities and denial of their reproductive rights, access to health facilities and political rights.

In the endline survey women were asked whether they had faced any form of violence in last 12 months preceding the survey and if they had, to what extent and by whom. Table 5.5a and Figure 5.3a present the types and perpetrators of the violence against women in the last 12 months preceding the survey. The survey reveals that the level of abuse is highest in Kishanganj (69%), followed by Kanpur (26%) but less than 10 per cent in the remaining districts, and is the lowest in Aizawl. Overall, there has been an increase in the reporting of violence against women in the endline survey as compared to baseline survey.

Table 5.5a

Percentage of women aged 13–24 who experienced any type of violence in the last 12 months and the perpetrators of violence

Type of violence and perpetrator	*Kanpur**	*Kishanganj*		*Bellary*		*Guntur*		*Aizawl*	
	EL (494)	*BL (539)*	*EL (465)*	*BL 488*	*EL 556*	*BL 472*	*EL 417*	*BL (471)*	*EL (439)*
Young women who experienced violence in the last 12 month	**25.5**	42.3	**68.6**	9.2	**4.5**	5.1	**8.2**	21.1	**1.4**
Type of violence experienced									
Pushed	**37.3**	14.5	**42.6**	1.6	**36.0**	0.4	**26.5**	7.9	**0.0**
Punched	**33.3**	11.9	**27.3**	1.2	**24.0**	1.9	**8.8**	11.5	**0.0**
Kicked	**16.7**	3.0	**11.3**	1.6	**36.0**	2.8	**17.6**	0.6	**0.0**
Others	**5.6**	12.9	**6.0**	4.7	**4.0**	0.0	**2.9**	1.1	**1.4**
Violence inflicted by									
Mother/mother-in-law	**31.0**	27.1	**31.7**	38.6	**32.0**	57.7	**12**	20.8	**0.0**
Father/father-in-law	**3.2**	16.4	**21.0**	24.4	**20.0**	32	**8.2**	27.7	**16.7**
Brother/sister	**20–6**	16.9	**24.8**	2.2	**16.0**	28	**2.9**	18.8	**0.3**
Husband/boyfriend	**33.3**	25.8	**29.8**	22.2	**44.0**	48	**8.8**	13.9	**33.3**
Other relatives/friends/neighbours	**20.6**	12.0	**6.3**	13.3	**16.0**	8	**70.6**	15.8	**50.0**
Total Women	**126**	225	**319**	44	**25.0**	26	**34**	101	**6**

* Information from the baseline survey is not presented due to change in intervention after the baseline survey.

The increase in reporting of domestic violence could be due to empowerment of women through awareness and recognition of such incidents over the period. CHARCA intervention to empower women could be a force that propels increase in reporting as many support systems like panchayat, police, NGOs, etc. were identified as resource groups in these districts to safeguard women's vulnerability.

Mostly, women are mistreated or beaten by their husbands/boyfriends (30–33%), followed by their mothers/mothers-in-law (31%) in Kanpur, Kishanganj and Bellary. However, in Guntur, 71 per cent of women reported being beaten by other relatives/friends/neighbours. In Aizawl also, 50 per cent of the women experience violence by persons other than close relatives, followed by 33 per cent who are beaten by their husbands/boyfriends.

Figure 5.3a

Violence against young women in CHARCA districts (%)

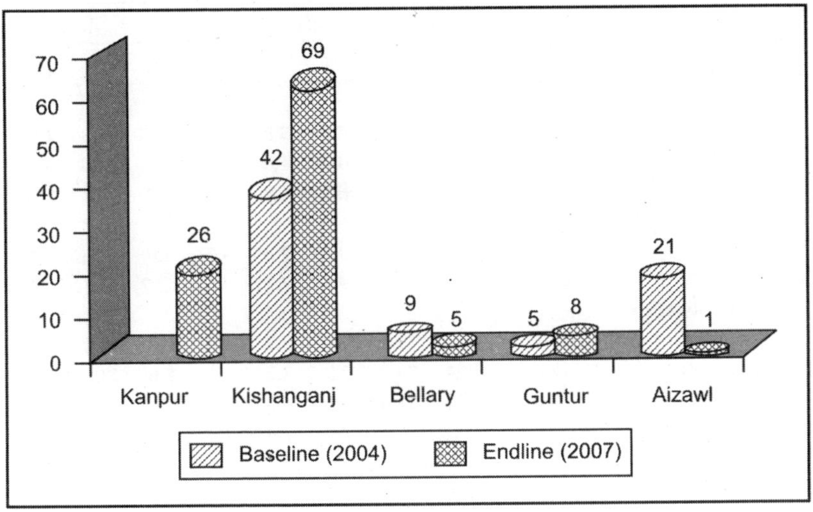

Figure 5.3b

Percentage of women reporting violence in the last 12 months (Panel Study)

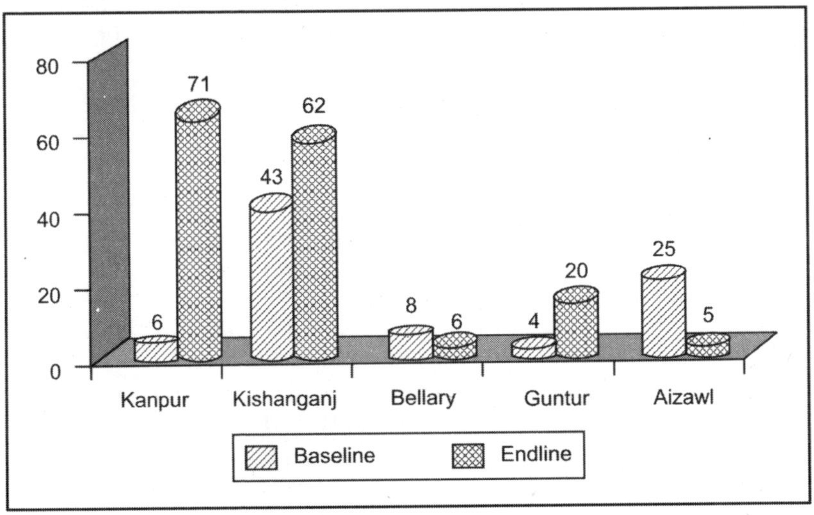

Table 5.5b

Prevalence of experience of violence among young women by selected background characteristics (%)

Background characteristics	*Kanpur**	*Kishanganj*		*Bellary*		*Guntur*		*Aizawl*	
	EL	*BL*	*EL*	*BL*	*EL*	*BL*	*EL*	*BL*	*EL*
Age (completed years)									
13–16	**19.2**	33.9	**67.3**	8.8	**3.3**	9.0	**16.5**	23.3	**2.6**
17–20	**22.6**	36.9	**65.2**	10.6	**4.3**	2.9	**7.7**	22.9	**0.6**
21–24	**36.4**	34.8	**72.3**	6.5	**6.0**	4.5	**3.7**	15.3	**1.4**
Marital Status									
Married	**33.7**	42.9	**73.4**	9.2	**7.3**	4.7	**4.0**	22.6	**1.4**
Unmarried	**21.0**	34.3	**63.0**	9.3	**2.1**	5.5	**13.7**	20.3	**1.4**
Women's Education									
Illiterate	**45.7**	36.8	**71.8**	9.8	**7.7**	6.1	**0.0**	33.3	**0.0**
<5 years complete	**50.0**	38.4	**73.3**	7.7	**3.3**	12	**7.6**	23.5	**0.0**
5–7 years complete	**27.0**	45.7	**61.4**	7.3	**6.3**	7.1	**10.5**	28.6	**2.3**
8–9 years complete	**27.6**	37.3	**69.6**	2.7	**2.4**	4.3	**9.7**	22.2	**0.7**
10 and above	**17.4**	26.2	**62.3**	17.3	**0.7**	1.9	**7.2**	20.8	**1.6**
Husband's Education									
Illiterate	**50**	59.6	**76.5**	0.0	**9.3**	5.3	**4.0**	100.0	**0.0**
<5 years complete	—	21.4	**79.1**	15.8	**0.0**	8.3	**9.5**	0.0	**0.0**
5–7 years complete	**56.3**	48.4	**68.0**	4.3	**9.3**	6.9	**6.3**	23.5	**0.0**
8–9 years complete	**35.3**	48.0	**80.0**	8.8	**0.0**	0.0	**0.0**	16.7	**5.6**
10 and above	**27.6**	46.7	**62.5**	3.5	**6.2**	2.7	**0.0**	21.9	**0.0**
Membership in CBOs									
Yes	**17.6**	20	**69.6**	22.7	**3.1**	4.3	**5.7**	22.4	**1.6**
No	**25.1**	38.2	**66.7**	8.6	**7.0**	5.2	**9.4**	18.5	**0**
Women's Occupation									
Homemaker	**25.1**	38.9	**66.9**	11.5	**2.4**	3.2	**8.0**	20.1	**1.2**
Working as labourer/family farm	**41.7**	31.6	**31.6**	6.4	**7.8**	8.1	**16.0**	22.0	**4.5**
Salaried/paid job	**0.0**	16.7	**16.7**	3.3	**6.5**	7.7	**0.0**	31.6	**0.0**
Migratory Status of Husband									
Non-migrant	**36.4**	38.7	**70.5**	8.9	**5.2**	5.1	**4.1**	20.9	**1.9**
Migrant	**28.6**	42.3	**78**	66.7	**10.4**	0.0	**3.6**	0.0	**0.0**
Exposure to Mass Media									
Yes	**23.6**	37.8	**65.1**	9.8	**4.8**	4.8	**8.2**	20.6	**1.4**
No	**40.7**	38.7	**73.2**	4.1	**1.8**	6.6	**7.7**	33.3	**0.0**
Total (N)	**25.5** **(126)**	42.3 (225)	**68.6** **(319)**	9.2 (44)	**4.5** **(25)**	5.1 (26)	**8.2** **(34)**	21.1 (101)	**1.4** **(6)**

*Information from the baseline survey is not presented due to change in intervention after the baseline survey.

The panel data shows that the experience of violence among young women has increased in Kanpur and Kishanganj by 54 per cent and 20 per cent respectively, while in the remaining districts violence in the last 12 months shows a decline of 87 per cent in Bellary, 75 per cent in Guntur and 2 per cent in Aizawl.

Prevalence of violence among women by selected background characteristics is presented in Table 5.5b. Kanpur and Bellary show increasing violence with age, whereas in Guntur it is the reverse, where younger women reported more such experiences. In Aizawl and Kishanganj there is no marked variation in experience of violence in the last 12 months with age of women. By marital status, it is observed that married women in the districts of Kanpur, Kishanganj and Bellary experienced more violence in comparison to the unmarried women. However, in Guntur, it is the unmarried women who are facing more violence. Nevertheless, in Aizawl, both married and unmarried women have suffered an almost equal extent of domestic violence.

'... women are facing violence more within their home than community, mostly the married women are facing this kind of abuse ... drinking habit of husband is mainly responsible for beating up wife in our community ...'

—Woman FGD, Bellary

'... I know a woman in my parental village who suffered a lot due to the dowry system, she is dumped by her in-laws due to not bringing any dowry ... now her situation is even worse at her natal family where brother harasses her a lot after the death of her parents ...'

—Woman KI, Kishanganj

'... when I am not ready for sex with my husband it does not make any difference for him ... he comes home and wants sex ... sometimes even if I am not feeling well I cant say no as I am afraid he will beat me up ...'

—Woman KI, Guntur

'... now the women are coming out and speaking up about the coercion they are facing in their day-to-day life .... .they are discussing and seeking for help ...'

—Man FGD, Aizawl

'... if wife is not listening to things or she is doing something which husband doesn't like ... he tells him for many times ... if she doesn't listen to him ... what is left then?... at that situation you can't blame a husband for beating or scolding his wife ...'

—Man KI, Kanpur

Educational attainment of women does not show any distinct variation in terms of experience of violence. However, it is found that women who are illiterate and those not having completed even five years of education are mainly the sufferers of violence in Kanpur, Kishanganj and Bellary compared to women who have completed 10 or more years of education in all the districts, except in Aizawl. Husband's education also does not reveal any clear picture in this regard.

Membership in CBOs/NGOs shows a negative relation with the experience of violence, as it is found that violence is lower among women who are members in the districts of Kanpur, Bellary and Guntur, but higher among women having membership in Kishanganj. Further, experience of violence in Kanpur, Guntur and Aizawl is more among women working as labourers or in family farms (42%, 16% and 5% respectively) than homemakers (25%, 8% and 1% respectively). The trend is the opposite in Kishanganj, where more homemakers experience violence (67%), followed by those working as labourers or on family farms (32%) and salaried or paid jobs (17%). In Bellary, women working as labourers face more violence (8%), followed by salaried (7%) and homemakers (2%).

The survey results further indicate that in Kanpur and Guntur, experience of violence is more felt by those women whose husbands are non-migrant, while women whose husbands are migrants have reported more violence in the districts of Kishanganj and Bellary. Similarly, with respect to exposure to mass media, prevalence of violence is higher among women not exposed to mass media in Kanpur and Kishanganj. However, in Bellary and Guntur women having mass media exposure have experienced more violence than others.

Violence against women has been an issue across cultures and societies. The dynamism of atrocity against women has always been apparent, irrespective of development of societies. The interlinkage of different socio-cultural and environmental factors is largely responsible for this social evil. The dynamism of the violence against women will be justified mainly through qualitative insights. In tune with survey findings, the qualitative data reveals the presence of atrocity in micro and community level across the five CHARCA districts, even after three years of intervention programmes intending to build the capacity of the marginalized gender.

The issue needs a long run dynamic programme design and contextual implementation. Conversely, there is evidence from different communities regarding the negation or normalization of atrocity against women and the increasing realization among men that of violence against women is a pathological behaviour.

Sexual violence against women

Men perceive marriage as the 'right' to unconditional sexual access and women do not have the right to say 'no' to conjugal sex. Therefore, forced sex within marriage is still not considered as rape. Population-based studies report between 12 and 25 per cent women experience attempted or compelled forced sex by an intimate partner or ex-partner at some point of time in their lives. CHARCA has attempted to capture the extent of sexual violence experienced by women from women's reporting of forced penetrative or coercive sex, especially within the context of marriage.

Figure 5.4

Women's experience of sexual violence (%)

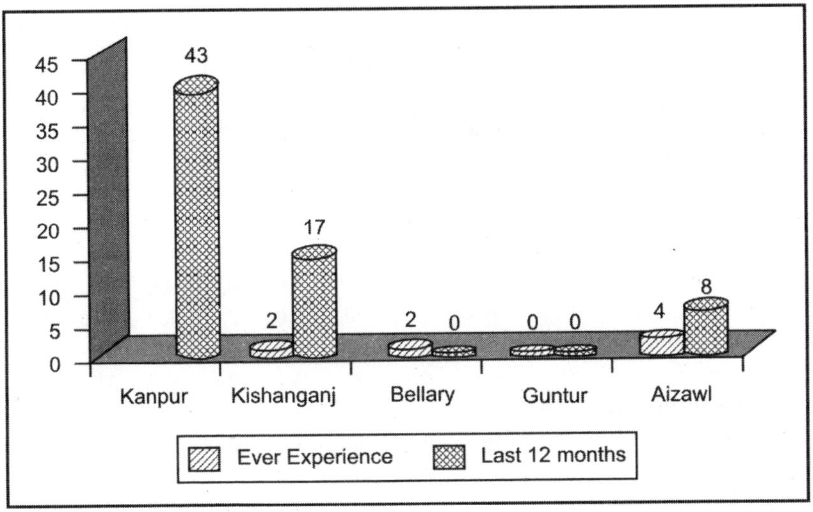

Table 5.5c and Figure 5.4 present sexual violence among young women by demographic and socio-economic characteristics. More women suffer sexual violence by almost all the background characteristics in the districts of Kanpur, Kishanganj and Bellary. It can be inferred that ever experience of sexual violence in Kanpur, and Bellary, and experience of sexual violence in last 12 months in Kanpur increases with an increase in women's age. Sexual violence in last 12 months is reported to be 100 per cent in Bellary among women aged 13–20 while it is 60 per cent among women aged 21–24. About 25 per cent and 20 per cent women aged 17–20 and 21–24 reported experience of sexual violence in Kishanganj and Aizawl respectively.

Table 5.5c

Percentage of women aged 13–24 who had ever experienced sexual violence

Background characteristics	*Kanpur*	*Kishanganj*		*Bellary*		*Guntur*			*Aizawl*
	Ever	*Last 12 months*	*Ever*	*Last 12 months*	*Ever*	*Last 12 months*	*Ever*	*Ever*	*Last 12 months*
Age (completed years)									
13–16	0.6	0.0	1.8	0.0	1.1	100.0	1.0	0.9	0.0
17–20	3.6	28.6	3.0	25.0	1.4	100.0	1.3	5.6	0.0
21–24	9.1	50.0	0.5	0.0	3.0	60.0	0.6	4.1	20.0
Marital Status									
Married	9.5	30.0	0.8	50.0	3.1	75.0	0.4	5.6	0.0
Unmarried	1.2	66.7	2.8	0.0	0.7	100.0	1.6	3.5	12.5
Women's Education									
Illiterate	8.7	66.7	1.8	33.3	2.4	50.0	0.0	0.0	0.0
<5 years complete	15.0	33.3	0.0	0.0	3.3	100.0	0.0	0.0	0.0
5–7 years complete	5.1	0.0	0.0	0.0	2.7	100.0	0.8	6.8	0.0
8–9 years complete	3.4	66.7	5.4	0.0	1.2	100.0	0.0	4.3	0.0
10 and above	2.7	0.0	3.3	0.0	0.0	0.0.0	2.2	3.1	16.7
Husband's Education									
Illiterate	0.0	0.0	0.0	0.0	4.2	60	0.0	0.0	0.0
<5 years complete	0.0	25.0	2.3	0.0	0.0	0.0	4.8	0.0	0.0
5–7 years complete	18.8	40.0	2.0	100.0	0.0	0.0	0.0	100.0	0.0
8–9 years complete	9.8	30.0	0.0	0.0	0.0	0.0	0.0	0.0	0.0
10 and above	9.2	0.0	0.0	0.0	4.6	100.0	0.0	3.8	0.0
Membership in NGOs/CBOs									
Yes	5.9	16.7	0.0	0.0	1.0	100.0	0.0	4.2	9.1
No	2.9	14.0	0.0	0.0	2.7	71.4	1.9	1.7	0.0
Women's Occupation									
Homemaker	4.3	30.8	1.6	20	1.2	75	0.9	3.9	9.1
Working as labourer/family farm	4.2	0.0	0.0	0.0	3.1	83.3	1.2	4.5	0.0
Salaried/paid job	0.0	0.0	10.0	0.0	0.0	0.0	0.0	0.0	0.0
Migratory Status of Husband									
Non-migrant	10.6	22.2	0.6	0.0	1.9	66.7	0.6	5.7	0.0
Migrant	7.1	10.5	2.0	100	4.7	80.0	0.0	16.7	0.0
Exposure to Mass Media									
Yes	3.6	37.5	1.7	25.0	1.8	77.8	0.7	3.9	8.3
No	9.3	60.0	1.7	0.0	1.8	100	7.7	0.0	0.0
Total (N)	**4.3**	**42.9**	**1.7**	**16.7**	**1.8**	**0.8**	**0.9**	**3.9**	**8.3**
	494	**21**	**465**	**6**	**556**	**10**	**417**	**439**	**12**

The ever experience of sexual violence is more among married women in Kanpur, Bellary and Aizawl, while in Kishanganj and Guntur it is higher among unmarried women. In the last 12 months sexual violence is reported more among married women in Bellary and Aizawl, but is higher among the unmarried women in Kanpur (67%) and Bellary (100%).

The survey also indicates sexual violence in last 12 months among all women with nine years of complete education in Bellary, and 67 per cent each among illiterate as well as having 8–9 years of completed education in Kanpur. Whereas in Bellary and Aizawl, experience of violence shows an inverse relationship with the educational attainment of women. Husband's education also does not show any distinct variation in the context of sexual violence against women. However, all women having 5–7 years complete education in Kishanganj and those having education of 10 or more years in Aizawl reported experience of sexual violence.

> '... while travelling in bus boys tease girls and from back side they also pull hair of girls or else they stick some posters to the back of girls. When we have special classes and it will be late to come to home at nights the boys tease in vulgar language at market places ...'
>
> —Woman FGD, Bellary
>
> '... There is a young girl who had committed suicide because her father had sexually assaulted her. Her mother was no more and she was helpless ...'
>
> —Woman KI, Kanpur
>
> '... its difficult for a single woman to walk in the evening alone on the street, even they don't spare passing a comment to a teenage girl if found alone ... all have a filthy attitude towards women ...'
>
> —Woman FGD, Kishanganj
>
> '... rape cases have come down in few years ... now girls are more aware and talking about any mistreatment...earlier they were keeping silent which was encouraging the men to perform the act again ... now girls are daring to expose the guilt ...'
>
> —Peer educator, FGD, Aizawl
>
> '... her cousin used to do all the bad things with her and it was all happening within home only ... when she told her family everybody blamed her character ... her cousin was encouraged by the silence of the family members and he used to do it often...one day she ran away from her home, nobody knows where she is now ...'
>
> —Woman KI, Guntur

Experience of sexual violence by CBO/NGO membership also shows mixed results, where it has been reported to be higher among women having membership in such organizations in Kanpur and Aizawl, while in Bellary it is higher among women not having membership. Similarly, women members of CBOs/NGOs have had more experience of sexual violence in Kanpur and this being 100 per cent in Bellary.

Women having no exposure to mass media reported more experience of sexual violence in Kanpur and Guntur while higher sexual violence in last 12 months is reported by women not having mass media exposure in the districts of Bellary and Kanpur. Further, it is found that the ever experience of sexual violence is higher among women whose husbands are migrants in the districts of Kishanganj (2% against 0.65%), Bellary (5% against 2%) and Aizawl (17% against 6%). In Kanpur violence is higher among women not having migrant husbands (10% against 7%). Sexual violence in last 12 months is reported to be higher among women having migrant husbands in Bellary (80% against 67%), while it is higher among women whose husbands are non-migrants in Kanpur (22% against 11%).

Experience of sexual violence among women by economic characteristics indicates that it is slightly more among those working as labourers or on family farms in Bellary, Guntur and Aizawl. Moreover, in Bellary, the experience of sexual violence in last 12 months is 7 per cent higher among labourers compared to the homemakers.

Physical versus sexual violence

The CHARCA endline survey also endeavoured to assess young women's vulnerability towards acquiring STI/HIV and other reproductive health problems as experienced due to the combinations of both physical and

Table 5.5d

Percentage of women aged 13–24 who had ever experienced physical or sexual violence

District	*Percentage who have experienced*			
	Physical violence	*Sexual violence*	*Physical or sexual violence*	*Physical and sexual violence*
Kanpur	25.5	4.3	26.5	3.2
Kishanganj	68.6	1.7	100.0	2.5
Bellary	4.5	1.8	4.5	1.8
Guntur	8.2	1.0	8.4	0.7
Aizawl	1.4	3.9	5.2	0.0

sexual abuse. Table 5.5d shows the variation in ever experience of sexual violence by young women in endline survey. Violence against women is mostly inflicted in the districts of Kishanganj and Kanpur. Twenty-five per cent of women experience physical and another 26 per cent either physical or sexual violence in Kanpur. In Kishanganj all the women reported physical or sexual violence, and 69 per cent physical violence alone. Similarly, in Bellary (5% each) and Guntur (8% each), most women reported physical violence or either of physical or sexual violence. In Aizawl, besides more women reporting physical or sexual violence, some women experience solely sexual violence (4%). Clearly, physical violence or either physical or sexual violence is mostly reported by women in Kishanganj and Kanpur, whereas sexual violence is more prevalent in Bellary and Aizawl. Moreover, women who reported both physical and sexual violence are more in Kanpur, closely followed by Kishanganj and Bellary.

Community level support for women

The existence of an effective support system such as police, panchayat and nari adalats or CBOs/NGOs and mahila mandals are crucial for women experiencing violence or abuse to provide necessary help and guidance. Women who had experienced violence were asked about any support they sought from any formal or informal sources.

Table 5.6

Percentage of women aged 13–24 who had experienced violence and sought support in the last 12 months

Types of support system	*Kanpur**	*Kishanganj*		*Bellary*		*Guntur*		*Aizawl*	
	EL	*BL*	*EL*	*BL*	*EL*	*BL*	*EL*	*BL*	*EL*
Formal sources of support†	0.8	4.2	8.5	0.0	0.0	2.2	0.2	1.6	0.0
Informal sources of support‡	0.4	8.3	6.9	42.3	1.8	15.6	4.1	8.4	0.2
Experienced violence	25.5	42.3	68.6	9.2	4.5	5.1	8.2	21.1	1.4

* Information from the baseline survey is not presented due to change in intervention after the baseline survey.

† Police, Nari Adalat, Panchayat, Health Centre.

‡ CBO/NGO, Mahila Mandal, Peers.

Among women experiencing violence, those seeking any formal support such as police, panchayat or nari adalat, ranges from less than 1 per cent in Guntur and Kanpur to 9 per cent in Kishanganj, which also shows a 4 per cent increase compared to the baseline survey (Table 5.6, Figure 5.5). The situation of seeking support from any informal source is also not encouraging as the proportion varies from less than 1 per cent in Aizawl and Kanpur, to 2 per cent in Bellary, 4 per cent in Guntur and 7 per cent in Kishanganj. In Kanpur and Kishanganj, women's seeking formal support has increased slightly than from informal sources. In Guntur women prefer informal source for support against violence inflicted on them. There has been an overall decline in seeking informal support, varying from 40 per cent in Bellary to around 10 per cent in Guntur, Kanpur and Aizawl and 3 per cent in Kishanganj.

Figure 5.5

Percentage of women reporting type of support in case of violence

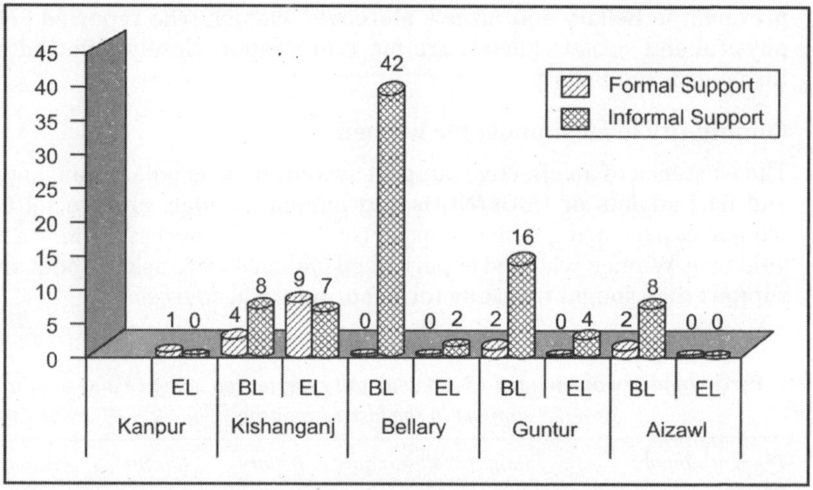

Providing and facilitating support system for different problems and issues and enabling community to avail the support platform is an uphill task, particularly in case of violence and abuse which is deeply rooted in gender roles. Although the survey shows a varying result for formal and informal support system across the five districts, the qualitative findings show the potentiality of informal support system in a rural structure where informal groups are more powerful. The pattern definitely shows the programme revitalizing the local informal support system as a sustainable platform of intervention.

Conclusions

- The contribution of CHARCA in reducing violence against women is evident. The programmes and activities of the women information centre have not only enhanced the reporting of violence

'... where to go for complaining about the abusing behaviour which happens at home ... the officers are not doing there own work, why they will come to solve my home problem and how I can expect that they will be honest with me while I don't have any right in my own home and can't bribe them ...'

—Woman KI, Kanpur

'... It is often seen that women in our community are holding meetings and talking about the problems they face at home and they also intervene directly in each other's problems in a group. It is found to be very effective in changing the attitude of the husbands towards their wives at a village set-up ...'

—Man FGD, Bellary

'... if the mistreatment against any woman comes to the knowledge of the senior persons of our villages they will surely probe into the case, and put sanctions on the husband for beating his wife. It has been happened in the past in our village which certainly impacts the behaviour of men in our village ...'

—Man KI, Guntur

'... there are some instances of police's non-cooperation towards the victimized women ... one such woman in our village has gone to complain against her in-laws in police ... nothing happened to them ... it resulted in deserting the woman by her husband and his family ... now she is staying alone in another village with lots of difficulties ...'

—Woman KI, Kishanganj

'... we came to know about the situation of a woman who used to beaten up by her father in this community ... we intervened and talked to her father... initially he was angry and was adamant by his stand, he was having a complaint of not having a son ... we keep on talking and talking and showing instances of success of other girls around his community ... now he has changed a lot ... planning to send his daughter for studies ...'

—Peer educator, FGD, Aizawl

but also issues discussed in CBO/NGO meetings. There is ample evidence of an increase in women's awareness and collective actions in opposing violence against women which cuts across all the CHARCA districts.

- The proportion of women who needed husband's permission to visit healthcare services has declined almost in all districts except Kishanganj, and 'to visit natal family' declined in all districts except Bellary and Kishanganj. The proportion of women who do not need husband's permission to visit neighbourhood has considerably increased in all districts except in Kishanganj. However, for participating in CBO/NGO meetings, the need for permission has declined in all districts except in Bellary.

- The perception that husbands should be accepted if they have extra-marital relations has also declined significantly. However, the difference is not significant between members and non-members of CBOs/NGOs. Similarly, the percentage of young women who reported that they do not have the ability to refuse sex if they are not willing has declined in all districts. In the endline survey, a significant proportion of women who have membership reported to have the ability to refuse sex compared to non-members, except in Kishanganj.
- Incidence of violence are highest in Kishanganj, followed by Kanpur. Incidence of violence in Kanpur and Bellary increase with age, while in Guntur more younger women experienced violence. In Aizawl and Kishanganj, there has been no marked variation in the experience of violence in the last 12 months. Married women in Kanpur, Kishanganj and Bellary have reported more violence in comparison to the unmarried women. However, in Guntur, more unmarried women reported violence. In Aizawl, both married and unmarried women experienced violence in the same extent. In Kanpur all women who are not currently married but were earlier married at some point of time have experienced violence.
- Membership of CBCs/NGOs shows a negative relationship with the experience of violence, as reports of violence are lower among women who are members, as indicated in Kanpur, Bellary and Guntur. But, in Kishanganj, reporting of violence is higher among women having membership.
- Sexual violence against women is also the highest among young women in Kanpur, Kishanganj and Bellary. Experience of sexual violence exhibits an inverse relationship with educational attainment in Kanpur, Aizawl and Bellary. Also, experience of both ever and recent sexual abuse is higher in urban areas and among women working as labourers in Bellary.
- The proportion of women seeking support, both formal and informal, is highest in Kishanganj, which also marks a slight increase in the case of formal support sought. Moreover, women seeking support from informal sources has shown an overall decline – highest in Bellary (40%) and about 10 per cent in Guntur, Kanpur and Kishanganj.

6

Prevalence of STIs and the Responsiveness of Healthcare Services

Understanding the dynamics of sexual and reproductive health problems among young women in terms of sexually transmitted infections (STIs) and the responses by the healthcare system is an apparent reason to arrest the bulgy infections, including HIV. Globally, as well as in India, reproductive and sexual health problems show an increasing share in the burden of diseases over the recent years. Most intervention policies advocate for synergizing the sexual health component with the other packages of action programmes for curbing the pandemic and to ensure an enabling environment for the marginalized core groups.

As observed in recent past, nearly half of new HIV infections worldwide occurred among the youth aged 15–29 years, which suggests the need to address their sexual behaviours. As in 2005, STIs, including HIV mainly affect sexually active young people, accounting for 32 per cent of AIDS cases reported in India and the number of young women living with HIV/AIDS is twice that of young men (NACO, 2005).

Studies on various interventions have shown increase in safe sex, either through condom use or avoiding penetrative sex, among the young people. However, a study has indicated that as many societies in developing countries tend to be more conservative or traditional, strategies such as giving condoms free of charge and providing information through school talks and leaflets, even in communities with high awareness of HIV/AIDS or sex-related diseases have shown disappointing results. The study also brings out how the qualitative research has emerged as a valuable method to understand the 'community perspective' that shapes sexual behaviours and helps in explaining why providing information and condoms – while important – are often not enough to change behaviours and how they might be improved (Marston and King, 2006).

Studies have cited diverse causes of the increased rates of STIs/HIV in young people but the main reasons include biological factors, risky sexual behaviour patterns (early initiation of sex, pre-marital sex, bi-sexual orientation and multiple sexual partners), transmission dynamics and treatment-seeking behaviour (Harms et al., 1998). In general, studies have indicated that women have a higher incidence of STIs than men because of their greater biological susceptibility. The present dearth of STI education in India is a major concern, particularly in schools (UNFPA, 2004).

Decrease in the sexual health problems within a vulnerable community over a period of time definitely indicates a programme's efficacy for not only fighting back the HIV but also empowering the marginalized target population. Against this backdrop the current study assesses the change in the trend of STIs within the communities, pattern of treatment-seeking behaviour, quality of services available across the five CHARCA districts, along with an in-depth look into the cultural dynamics of the infections.

Self-reported symptoms of STIs by young women

Recent research evidence shows that symptom-based reporting of STIs not only indicates the prevalence of the different STDs, but also measures the individual and community level perception and attitude towards STIs. In the endline study, young women were asked whether they had experienced any one of the nine symptoms of STIs mentioned during the last 12 months. Except Bellary, in the remaining three districts, there has been a decrease in reporting of at least one symptom of STI among young women between the baseline and endline survey. Reporting of any STI among young women in Bellary has slightly increased from 23 per cent in the baseline to 28 per cent in the endline study. This could possibly reflect the enhancing awareness and the ability to recognize the STI symptoms as a problem among young women in Bellary, rather than normalizing which might be credited to different awareness programmes. In Aizawl, where education level is already high among the young women due to different socio-historical factors, the prevalence of self-reported symptoms has decreased significantly from three-fourth in baseline study to less than one-fourth in the recent endline study. The trend is somewhat similar in the case of other three districts reflecting the credibility to CHARCA intervention programmes. The prevalence of self-reported symptoms has decreased from 85 per cent to 62 per cent in Kishanganj and from 28 per cent to 16 per cent in Guntur since the baseline survey (Figure 6.1).

Figure 6.1

Percentage of young women having at least one symptom of STI

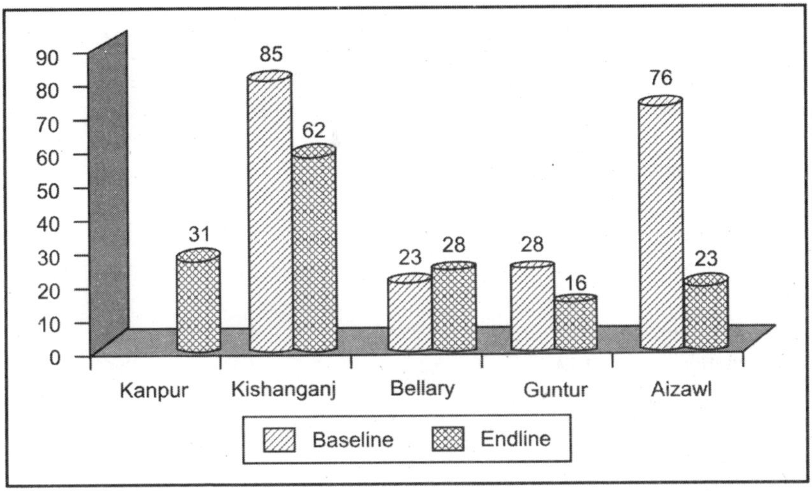

In symptom-based reporting, it is always important to look at the issue symptom-wise for better scientific legitimacy. Table 6.1 presents the symptom-wise prevalence of self-reported STIs across the five CHARCA districts with a comparative picture of these nine symptoms of STIs between the baseline and endline survey. It is quite evident that of the nine symptoms asked, eight symptoms show a decreasing trend in all the districts except Bellary. The self-reported symptom as, 'some mass coming out of vagina' shows an increasing trend in Kishanganj and Bellary. In Kishanganj and Bellary too the percentage of women reporting 'some mass coming out of vagina' has increased from 8 per cent in the baseline survey to ten per cent in the endline survey and 4 per cent in the baseline survey to 13 per cent in the endline survey respectively. The proportion of women reporting each of nine symptoms has increased in Bellary. Judging from the changing trend observed across the time period as indicated by indicators like education and source of awareness among young women in Bellary, it can be safely assumed that the CHARCA awareness programme has effected to better reporting of STI symptoms in Bellary.

Table 6.1

Percentage of women reporting different symptoms of STIs during the last 12 months in the five CHARCA districts

Symptoms of STI	*Kanpur**	*Kishanganj*		*Bellary*		*Guntur*		*Aizawl*	
	EL (494)	*BL (539)*	*EL*	*BL (488)*	*EL*	*BL (472)*	*EL (417)*	*BL (471)*	*EL (439)*
Itching over vulva	9.3	31.8	6.7	1.2	4.3	3.2	3.8	29.4	2.5
Boils/ulcers/warts around vulva	10.5	41.3	7.7	0.6	1.8	1.5	0.0	4.3	0.0
Pain during sexual intercourse	3.4	15.2	5.4	1.0	5.0	4.1	2.9	5.7	0.7
Swelling in the groin	0.8	24.8	5.6	0.4	1.8	0.6	2.6	2.1	0.0
Difficulty/pain while urinating	2.0	26.4	22.2	2.9	5.6	2.8	2.4	17.0	0.7
Frequent urination	4.5	23.8	19.6	3.3	6.1	4.7	1.2	39.4	5.5
Itching/irritation around genital	14.4	14.1	6.2	0.0	3.6	2.6	2.6	20.0	1.6
Some mass coming out of vagina	7.3	8.0	9.5	3.5	13.1	9.6	1.9	29.1	15.5
Escape of urine while coughing or sneezing	0.4	11.0	11.2	0.0	0.5	0.2	0.0	8.7	0.5
Having at least one symptom	48.4	85.2	94.4	23.0	55.6	27.5	37.2	75.6	27.1

* Information from the baseline survey is not presented due to change in intervention area after the baseline survey.

Further, the most commonly reported symptoms, 'itching over vulva', 'swelling over groin' and 'pain during sexual intercourse', with a variance across the districts, have decreased over the three-year time period (2004–2007). Reporting of 'pain during sexual intercourse' in Kanpur is 3 per cent in the endline survey. This has declined in Kishanganj from 25 per cent in the baseline to 6 per cent in the endline survey, in Bellary from 4 per cent in the baseline to 3 per cent in endline survey, and in Aizawl from 6 per cent in the baseline to less than 1 per cent in endline survey.

Symptom like 'itching over vulva', which is reported by a large proportion of young women in Kishanganj and Aizawl (32% and 29% respectively), has significantly decreased in the endline study (7% and 3% respectively). The decrease reflects the translation of knowledge about menstrual and sexual hygiene into practice. Similarly, with 'boils/ulcers/warts around vulva' which is an apparent infection sign also shows a decreasing trend in Kishanganj from 41 per cent in the baseline survey to 8 per cent in the endline survey, in Guntur from 2

'... earlier I have not seen anybody talking on such issues in our village or in the community ... now we can find girls getting together, holding meetings regularly ... discussing the issues like sexual health and HIV, which we were considering filthy, helping each other for getting the right knowledge.'

—Man KI, Kanpur

'... we are talking frankly about the symptoms of the health problems and make sure that the young girls are comfortable enough to share all their problems with us ... we also ensure that some one who gets this kind of problem, should get treatment free form government hospitals ... we follow it up without missing a single ...'

—Peer educator, FGD, Kishanganj

'... people of this community have started coming out with the symptoms ... though they there is some overreporting of symptoms, still it is good thing that people are getting aware about the STIs and HIV and they are thinking of sharing the problem freely which is a positive sign ...'

—Public health service provider,
interviewed within Man KI, Bellary

'... my wife used to talk about the sexual health problems and how important it is to take care of and make treatment at correct time ... she knows more than me ...'

—Man KI, Aizawl

'... how you will control the men ... they are going whatever available to them and its very easy in our place ... you go to market or bus stand, pay 50 rupees and get a woman ... this kind of behaviour should be checked else you have to welcome the STDs and even HIV ...'

—Man KI, Guntur

per cent in the baseline survey and none in the endline survey, and in Aizawl 4 four per cent the in baseline survey to none in the endline.

The qualitative findings reflect the in-depth sights into the issue of sexual health problems among young women. Although the associating factors and outcomes vary from district to district, the marginalized status of women is found to be a common under force which drives the intermediary variables in tune with current socio-cultural settings. Apart from the above common symptoms shown in Table 6.1, in most of the FGDs 'white discharge' is mentioned as another experienced symptom across the districts. The survey findings of declining prevalence of STIs are being supported by the different levels of qualitative insights. Across the districts the programme has helped to break the culture of silence about sexual health problems. Different awareness strategies and direct health intervention programmes on a one-to-one outreach by the peer educators effort to counsel and encourage young women to avail treatment and proper management have benefited the community. The peer educators could desensitize and normalize the talk about sexual health problems among the young people.

The factors affecting the infections among young women remain almost similar across the five districts. Apparently cultural change has not happened over the three years' period, which of course is a short period to expect any drastic change in the age-old cultural practices. A wide range of factors that affect women's vulnerability are poverty-driven low paid sex work in Bellary, Guntur and Kanpur, the extent of pre-marital sexual encounter in Aizawl and the low socio-economic status of women in Kishanganj. Not only these factors affect women's sexual well-being, and minimize their sexual negotiation power, the rampant alcoholism among men in districts like Bellary and Guntur further endangers the scenario.

Characteristics of young women reporting STIs

While discussing the changing trend of STIs among a community, it is important to look at each character for getting a clearer picture of the programme efficacy. Table 6.2 shows distribution of women reporting of having at least one symptom of STI by their socio-demographic characteristics in the five districts. The baseline study across all the five districts shows that the prevalence of reported symptoms of STIs are positively related to age, marital status, education, membership of CBOs/ NGOs and exposure to mass media. In the endline study, the prevalence of self-reported symptoms of STIs shows some variations with age, membership and marital status.

The younger cohort in Aizawl has experienced the highest decline (87% change) in self-reported STIs, whereas in Kishanganj women in younger cohort experienced 43 per cent decline in reporting. The decline is only 4 per cent in Guntur. Within the educational categories, the decline in the proportion of women among higher educational category and low educated women does not show any significant change. It is apparent that the CHARCA intervention has equally benefited the women across the educational categories on sexual health matters.

Table 6.2

Percentage of young women having at least one symptom of STIs during last 12 months by some selected background characteristics in the five CHARCA districts

Background characteristics	*Kanpur**	*Kishanganj*		*Bellary*		*Guntur*		*Aizawl*	
	EL	*BL*	*EL*	*BL*	*EL*	*BL*	*EL*	*BL*	*EL*
Age (completed years)									
13–16	21.2	78.8	45.5	16.8	22.5	18.8	11.3	66.1	6.1
17–20	28.7	87.5	59.8	22.6	27.1	31.7	20.5	77.1	26.0
21–24	45.5	89.9	73.3	28.1	34.7	30.1	14.0	81.3	31.8
Marital Status									
Married	45.6	91.3	74.2	29.9	37.5	31.9	16.6	84.5	20.2
Unmarried	23.5	80.6	47.9	13.2	19.4	22.5	14.8	73.6	36.1
Women's Education									
Illiterate	47.8	85.8	71.8	30.1	41.1	27.8	7.7	100.0†	0.0
<5 years complete	55.0	89.3	61.1	21.2	25.0	36.0	21.2	76.5	50.0
5–7 years complete	28.8	81.6	70.5	22	24.3	26.2	21.0	76.0	9.1
8–9 years complete	29.7	83.6	42.9	17.8	14.6	28.3	11.3	74.2	15.2
10 years and above	27.2	81.6	41.0	14.8	23.7	26.8	12.2	75.9	29.1
Membership in NGOs/CBOs									
Yes	11.8	50.0	69.6	36.4	28.9	31.9	16.5	79.6	24.7
No	37.5	85.6	33.3	22.3	35.0	26.8	15.1	70.3	10.3
Exposure to Mass Media									
Yes	18.5	84.2	66.7	22.8	21.4	27.5	15.4	75.4	0.0
No	32.7	88.6	60.3	24.5	28.6	27.6	15.8	100.0	22.8
Total	31.2	85.2	61.9	23.0	27.9	27.5	15.8	75.6	22.8
Respondents	494	539	465	488	556	472	417	471	43.9

* Information from the baseline survey is not presented due to change in intervention after the baseline survey.

† Less than five cases.

In Kishanganj the prevalence of self-reported symptoms has declined more among unmarried women than married women. The pattern is reverse in case of Guntur and Aizawl. In Guntur the married women reported a higher decline of 48 per cent compared to unmarried women (34%). Similarly, in Aizawl, the married women reflected a 76 per cent decline in selfreported symptoms of STIs compared with unmarried women (51%).

To get a better comparative picture of the currently discussing issue and its correlates, 471 women who were interviewed in the baseline survey were followed up in the endline survey. The same issues like self-reporting, treatment seeking and quality of care were explored. The panel data reveals somewhat a similar trend with the cross-sectional results. There is a sharp decline in reporting of almost all symptoms of sexually transmitted infections except 'frequent urination' among the young women in the five CHARCA districts. A glance at the prevalence of any STIs indicates a favourable trend in relation to programme efficacy in curbing the infection rate (Figure 6.2). However, Bellary shows a different pattern than that of cross-sectional data. The fall in prevalence of any STI in Bellary is found to be significant in the panel data whereas the trend was found to be slightly higher in the cross-sectional data. It gives an impression that the intervention in this district is focused on a particular community with a programmatic bias.

Figure 6.2

Prevalence of at least one symptom of STIs among women in panel study

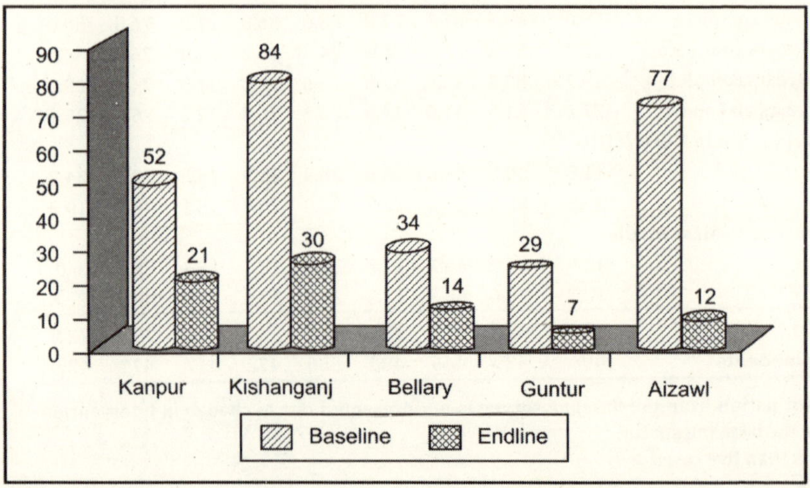

The gap between STI prevalence in cross-sectional and panel data indicates the need for even-intervention of any programme.

Self-reported symptoms of STIs among men

Men's reproductive and sexual health is equally vital to address the overall sexual and reproductive health well-being of a community. It is evident that men are the major source of channelizing the infection to women, who are either their spouse or casual partners of sex. The scenario of male sexual health is comparatively dicier in the Indian cultural context. Interface of perceived male gender, stigma attached to sexual issues make the discussion of male infection to be undercover. The culture of silence impedes male involvement, which no doubt is an important concern in managing the hazards of the infection among both women and men. The programme reach of men's perception, attitude and behaviour regarding STIs is another parameter that evaluates the efficacy of the intervention. Young men aged 15 to 29 were therefore asked about their perception, attitude and management of STIs.

Table 6.3

Percentage of men reported symptoms of STIs, including urethritis, during the last 12 months in the five CHARCA districts

Symptoms of STI	*Kanpur**	*Kishanganj*		*Bellary*		*Guntur*		*Aizawl*	
	EL	*BL*	*EL*	*BL*	*EL*	*BL*	*EL*	*BL*	*EL*
Pain during urination	6.8	25.6	10.4	17.6	5.4	17.6	32.7	13.4	4.9
Pain during sexual intercourse	2.8	16.6	2.4	1.2	3.2	1.2	3.7	1.5	0.0
Involuntary passing of semen	0.6	26.6	1.5	0.8	1.3	0.8	3.7	26.1	12
Abscess in penis	1.9	8.0	1.8	1.6	1.6	1.6	0.5	3.5	0.0
Wounds/sores	7.8	17.0	6.1	0.4	1.6	0.4	2.3	47.0	1.6
Yellowish/greenish discharge with smell from penis	0.6	3.5	1.2	1.6	0.6	1.5	0.9	2.0	0.0
Total	322	291	328	256	317	264	214	220	184

* Information from the baseline survey is not presented due to change in intervention after the baseline survey

Table 6.3 presents the picture of the self-reported symptomatic prevalence of STIs among young men in the five programme districts.

Except Guntur, the rest three districts are experiencing an overall decline in the symptomatic prevalence of STIs among young men. The most frequently mentioned symptoms across the five districts are 'pain during urination' and 'involuntary passing of semen'. The symptom 'yellowish discharge with smell from penis' (urethritis) has shown a decline in Kishanganj (4% in baseline and 1% in endline), Bellary (2% in baseline and 1% in endline), Guntur (2% in baseline and 1% in endline) and in Aizawl (2% in baseline and none in the endline).

Unlike women, reporting on sexual health problems, among young men shows a varying trend and prevalence across the five

'why to make such a big issue about men's sexual health problem, it is not that complicated ... most of them is physical structure disorder ... or due to some bad practice in childhood ... this all can be corrected by some practiced method which runs from ages in our villages and old people know about it ...'

—Man KI, Kishanganj

'... condom is a common factor among youths ... they don't hesitate even holding and making fun in public ... it was very uncommon feature in our time ... controlling today's young people's behaviour is difficult ... they should be aware for safety in their behaviour. And it is a good thing that they are getting aware of safety measures ...'

—Man KI, Bellary

'... I have heard from my friends discussing about the sexual health problems and how it is communicable. They are regular attendees of health meetings organized in our community ... we all should know about it. Knowledge can save lives ...'

—Man KI, Guntur

'... earlier the young girls were holding a shy figure and were not talking about this matter in meetings and other gatherings we organize in village, gradually they are showing much interest and even initiating the awareness programmes in their respective villages ...'

—Peer educator FGD, Kanpur

'... we used to organize meetings on talking about sexual health problems, its management and try to bring more and more people to the meetings ... men in our community are well aware of the sexual health problems and how to take care of it them. Talking about condom is a very common phenomenon in our community ...'

—Man KI, Aizawl

districts. The variation can be due to the main focus of the programme on womenfolk, which may have sidelined the young men through out the programme.

While probing further on the issue of male STIs, it was found that apart from the reported symptoms during the survey phase, performance-related symptoms like early ejaculation, structure of penis and semen-related symptoms like colour and thickness of semen were also discussed during focus group discussions (FGDs) among young men. Although there was a reflection on gender regarding sexual health problems, a sizeable number of discussions and interviews revealed the sensitization of young men across the five CHARCA districts. Interestingly, it is found that in districts like Bellary, Kanpur and Aizawl the messages regarding gender sensitization, healthcare and other information get diffused from the young women of those communities. Though it is not largely seen across the communities it is a positive sign of breaking ice and begin inter-gender dialogues particularly on health and gender issues in rural set-ups. The qualitative findings also support the declining prevalence of STIs among men in majority of the districts by justifying the growing awareness of condom use, rights-based approach to management and increasing discussions on sexual health issues among men at different platforms.

However, the threat of endangering the male sexual health and male sexual behavioural patterns in all the districts are felt and expressed in the discussions through FGDs and key informant interviews. Comparing the baseline findings, the sexual encounters and sexual intimacy have increased though in a low volume. The changing sexual avenues have the potential to pose a threat in the long run for the sexual well-being of both the genders. For example, in Bellary, the shift of male labour force from agriculture to mining industry has opened the ground for women to work in agriculture, mostly as daily wage labourers. The physical distance of farms from villages, the feudalistic power dynamics of landlords over the labourers and the lack of sexual negotiation power of women have made the situation easy for the young men to gratify their sexual needs with these women agricultural labourers working in the fields. This kind of sexual encounter is mostly casual in nature. Although condom use is reflected to increase even in casual sexual encounters among young men, a regular assessment of the level of risk in the sexual behaviour of young men is advisable in such changing cultural networks.

Utilization of healthcare services for STIs among young women

Cutting down the STIs among women has been a major strategy to reduce HIV vulnerability across cultures. It not only directly indicates the healthy sexual life of a particular community but also used as an indicator for assessing women's sexual bargaining power and reproductive autonomy. The rising pre-intervention figure of self-reported STIs in baseline study in five CHARCA district was a challenge before the programme implementation and management, especially looking at the geographical distribution of the intervention areas. However, the lowering infection rate in these districts is an apparent evidence of programme efficacy in managing the STIs. Further, this point is being validated by the improved utilization of healthcare facilities for treating the STIs among the young women across the five districts (Table 6.4).

Table 6.4

Proportion of women who sought treatment for STI in different health facilities during the past 12 months in the five CHARCA districts

Place of last treatment	*Kanpur**	*Kishanganj*		*Bellary*		*Guntur*		*Aizawl*	
	EL	*BL*	*EL*	*BL*	*EL*	*BL*	*EL*	*BL*	*EL*
Government†	15.4	6.5	30.8	8.0	33.8	18.5	18.1	20.8	7.7
Private	9.2	32.7	46.7	36.6	22.8	27.7	16.4	13.2	5.1
AYUSH‡	0.0	3.5	0.0	1.8	0.0	1.5	0.0	0.8	0.0
Chemist/medical shop	28.6	24.0	47.6	1.8	14.3	9.2	9.5	15.7	0.0
Number of women sought treatment	42	459	141	112	260	130	50	356	20

* Information from the baseline survey is not presented due to change in intervention after the baseline survey.

† Government facility includes municipal hospitals, PHCs and sub-centres.

‡ AYUSH refers to Ayurveda, Unani, Sidha and Homeopathy.

The utilization, of government healthcare facilities has increased over the three years period significantly in all the districts, except Aizawl. In Kanpur the utilization of government hospitals is 15 per cent in the endline survey. In Kishanganj it has increased to 31 per cent in the endline from 7 per cent in the baseline survey, in Bellary to 34 per cent in the endline survey from 8 per cent. In Guntur, however, the utilization of government health care facility has remained unchanged. The comparative figures of utilization of government health system in

Guntur and Aizawl may be affected by the sharp decline in sexually transmitted infected women during the three years' period. The utilization of private healthcare providers has declined in almost all the districts except Kishanganj. In Aizawl the utilization of private healthcare has decreased by 60 per cent. Not a single woman has reported for availing treatment under AYUSH health care in all five CHARCA districts.

Both the cross-sectional and the panel data reveal the increase in the utilization of public healthcare providers for managing STIs (Figure 6.3). The young women's treatment-seeking pattern in the followed up communities is far better than the women covered in cross-sectional data collection phase. The increasing use of government health facility is more significant than in the cross-sectional data.

Figure 6.3

Percentage of women availing government healthcare systems for treating STIs in the panel study

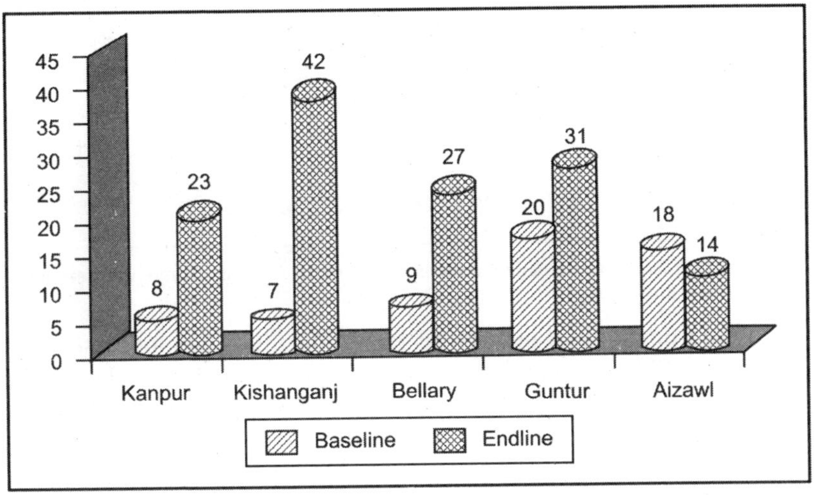

Further, the cross-sectional data of Guntur shows no change in the utilization of government healthcare system whereas in the panel data young women in Guntur reported more use of government health facilities for managing STIs. In the case of availing private healthcare system all the districts except Aizawl in the panel data have shown an increase whereas in cross-sectional study three out of four districts excluding Aizawl have shown a decline.

Utilization of healthcare services for STIs among young men

Addressing male sexual health problems is more sensitive and challenging to handle in any programme of intervention in the Indian cultural set-up. The determinants and associated factors have been discussed earlier. The pattern of STI management among the young men across the five CHARCA districts is showing a different pattern than that of women's. Except Bellary (38% in baseline to 65% in endline) and Kishanganj (3% in baseline to 12% in endline), in the other two districts, the utilization of government healthcare facilities for male STIs has declined across the time period.

Table 6.5

Proportion of men who sought treatment for STIs, in different health facilities during the past 12 months in the five CHARCA districts

Place of last treatment	*Kanpur**	*Kishanganj*		*Bellary*		*Guntur*		*Aizawl*	
	EL	*BL*	*EL*	*BL*	*EL*	*BL*	*EL*	*BL*	*EL*
Government	3.6	3.4	12.3	37.5	65.3	28.6	2.4	31.3	5.7
Private	5.5	32.2	8.9	18.8	24.1	64.3	22.4	8.1	5.7
AYUSH	0.0	4	0.0	43.8	0.0	0.0	0.0	0.0	0.0
Chemist/medical shop	1.8	15.4	9.6	0.0	0.0	7.1	4.7	10.1	0.0
Number of men sought treatment	6	149	24	32	26	14	25	99	4

* Information from the baseline survey is not presented due to change in intervention after the baseline survey.

The utilization of private healthcare facilities has increased only in Bellary (24% in endline from 19% in baseline). Similar to the baseline survey, the private health service providers are always popular among young men for treating STI symptoms in all the districts. The treatment seeking from AYUSH for STIs among young men showed a similar pattern as the young women. Not a single man has reported of treating STIs using AYUSH systems.

The infrequent treatment pattern for male STIs indicates the programmatic difficulties in mainstreaming young men in managing their sexual health problems in almost all the districts, except Bellary.

The qualitative insights regarding limitations in seeking men's healthcare indicate a different pattern to that of the survey findings. Most of the FGDs and key informants revealed that men are more worried about performance-related sexual illness rather than the

'... going to the government hospital is a risk for this kind of problems ... everything is kept in record ... any one can see for what problem you have gone ...'

—Young man FGD, Kanpur

'... I had a swelling in my penis tip for long ... I was into getting anyone who to talk about it and where to find out the treatment ... was trying my own home remedies and making the situation worse ... then one of my friends took me the hospital where I got cured ...'

—Man KI, Guntur

'... in our community earlier men were not ready to accept that the treatment is needed for any male sexual health problems... now they are coming out and convincing for treating the STIs ...'

—Peer educator, Bellary

'... my wife forced me to check it up by the doctor ... as she was in afraid that I got HIV ... I checked and got medicine for it ... it was just some infection in my growing nothing serious ... now I am fine ...'

—Man KI, Aizawl

'... these doctors give cheap medicine and only treat these problems ... they are specialized in treating sex diseases and you can find them in market places easily ...'

—Man KI, Kishanganj

symptomatic STIs. Private healthcare facilities are best preferred for sexual health problems. Most men depend on the untrained quacks and other unrecognized service providers who claim to treat effectively the sexual health problems. The anonymity, easy access and the problem-focused advertisements by these service providers are the major factors that influenced men across the five CHARCA districts for opting them.

Quality of care at the health facility last sought for STIs by women

Sustaining treatment-seeking behaviour, be it at the individual level or at the community level, largely depends on the quality of care provided by the healthcare givers. The experience and perception of individuals about the care providers and the facilities available determine selecting the healthcare provider. While talking about the sexual health seeking behaviour in a rural community, the interface of these factors in vital. Although many community-based programmes always work on bridging the gap between the healthcare seekers and vindicated healthcare providers, most of the time it becomes challenging to meet the objectives due to various administrative and logistic constraints. However, even the negative perceptions about the quality of care itself indicate the increasing awareness and critical evaluation of existing healthcare system.

As in the baseline survey, the women who have sought treatment either in government or private healthcare facilities were asked about their perceptions about seven components of quality of care. Table 6.6 shows the level of the quality of care available to the young women in five CHARCA districts over the time period.

Table 6.6

Percentage of women by their perception of quality of services for last treatment of STIs from public and private service providers during the past 12 months in the five CHARCA districts

Quality parameters	*Kanpur**	*Kishanganj*		*Bellary*		*Guntur*		*Aizawl*	
	EL	*BL*	*EL*	*BL*	*EL*	*BL*	*EL*	*BL*	*EL*
Availability of trained medical practitioner/doctor	21.6	41.0	71.6	70.5	19.6	33.0	73.6	47.3	93.3
Counselling	7.8	41.3	56.5	67.9	16.9	25.4	54.9	22.7	46.7
Availability of drugs	56.9	24.6	49.8	59	42.3	48.9	52.7	28.7	30.0
Physical examination	15.7	31.3	69.8	67.9	20.0	38.3	33	11.7	66.7
Follow-up was advised	9.8	35.3	65.3	56.4	3.1	25.9	16.5	18.6	80.0
Privacy	9.8	22.2	0.7	70.5	0.4	26.6	5.5	15.0	73.3
Adequate attention by service provider	0.0	14.6	0.4	69.2	0.0	14.9	1.1	26.7	93.3
Total	51	329	285	78	260	94	91	247	30

* Information from the baseline survey is not presented due to change in intervention after the baseline survey.

More young women in all four districts, except Bellary, reported availability of drugs in healthcare centres over the past three years. About the availability of a trained doctor, young women in Kishanganj (41% in baseline to 72% in endline) and in Guntur (33% in baseline to 74% in endline) reported a better situation compared to baseline survey. Except Aizawl, Kishanganj is the only district where components like counselling (41% in baseline and 57% in endline), physical examination (31% in baseline and to 65% in endline) and follow-up advice (35% in baseline and 65% in endline) are reported to have improved. However, none of these components of quality of care shows a consistent pattern across the five districts.

Components like privacy and adequate attention by the service provider, which are considered as the most important quality components while talking about the sexual health, show a sharp decline in all the districts except Aizawl. The growing number of patients and overcrowding at healthcare centres might be one of the causes behind lack of privacy and inadequate attention of service providers, resulting in poor perception about quality of care in reproductive and sexuai health services.

The panel results about the quality of care in five CHARCA districts have not revealed any difference than that of the cross-sectional. The availability of trained doctors has increased in Kishanganj (38% to 63%) and in Aizawl (49% to 81%). The rest of three districts show a decline in the availability of trained doctors and quality components like counselling and adequate attention by service providers. However, similar to cross-sectional data, 'availability of drugs' has shown an improvement in the five CHARCA districts, varying with a positive change of 21 per cent in Aizawl. The difficulties before any community-based intervention programme in changing the existing system which is governed by a completely different entity is well discussed earlier in this chapter, which can be seen as a justification for the arbitrary variation in quality of care components over the time period.

STIs and women's capacity

It is evident that awareness about condom is one of the indicators for controlling sexually infectious risks. An attempt has therefore been made to find the factors associated with awareness regarding condom, autonomy in decision-making regarding healthcare seeking, attitude towards husband's extra-marital relations and the capacity to refuse sex among the women having at least one symptom of STIs.

Table 6.7 shows a similar pattern with that of the baseline study. Knowledge about getting at least one source of acquiring male condoms has no impact on reducing the risk of getting STIs, except in Kishanganj. In Kishanganj, while 45 per cent of women who know at least one source of getting male condoms are reporting to have one of the symptoms of STI, 55 per cent young women who do not know a single source of getting male condoms are infected. In case of the knowledge of correct use of condom, the result is also in the same direction as the previous indicator. The women who are aware about the benefits of correct use of condom and knowing a place to get condom are more likely to be with at least one symptom of STIs.

Table 6.7

Percentage of women with at least one symptom of STIs during the last 12 months by extent of awareness about male condom

Background characteristics		*Kanpur**	*Kishanganj*		*Bellary*		*Guntur*		*Aizawl*	
		EL	*BL*	*EL*	*BL*	*EL*	*BL*	*EL*	*BL*	*EL*
Sources to get male condom	Does not know any location	27.6	84.4	55.4	23.2	23.6	23.2	12.9	70.4	6.7
	At least one location is known	72.4	85.0	44.6	21.1	76.4	44.3	87.1	82.7	93.3
Correct use of condom Can prevent STI infection	Yes	67.0	85.9	56.7	12.0	93.1	23.9	92.9	79.3	100.0
	No	1.3	91.1	18.5	10.7	6.9	28.6	0.6	69.6	0.0
	Don't know	7.9	90.0	7.5	27.7	0.0	27.9	0.0	66.4	0.0

* Information from the baseline survey is not presented due to change in intervention after the baseline survey.

Apparently there is no expected relationship between the condom awareness and prevalence of STIs among the young women. The contrast may owe to the fact that increasing awareness among young women resulted from the infections and discussions on its management. Against this backdrop one can safely assume that the knowledge and awareness among women who are suffering from STIs is increasing significantly.

In case of decision about healthcare utilization, the women who reported that their husbands are the sole authority to take decision about their health seeking behaviour, are found to suffer less from any kind of STIs than the women who take decision jointly. The possible justification might be husband's involvements in managing wife's sexual health problems, which is a healthy sign of changing gender dynamics.

More women who do not accept husband's extra-marital relationship and not having the ability to refuse sex have at least one symptom of STIs. The reason might be that, after getting infected the women remain in contact with the programmes and other interventions at different levels. Further, they may be aware of their own sexual and reproductive rights. On the other hand, it can be argued that, as women are already aware about their sexual rights and sexual health through other programmes, the reporting of symptoms of STIs is better.

Table 6.8

Percentage of women with at least one symptom of STIs during the last 12 months by some selected dimensions of reproductive and sexual rights

Reproductive and sexual rights matters		*Kanpur**	*Kishanganj*		*Bellary*		*Guntur*		*Aizawl*	
		EL	*BL*	*EL*	*BL*	*EL*	*BL*	*EL*	*BL*	*EL*
Utilization of health services should be decided	Jointly	92.1	79.0	58.3	24.4	27.5	24.9	88.4	73.8	75.8
	Husband only	3.8	77.8	10.3	11.1	27.8	50.0	1.9	86.8	2.4
	Wife only	3.8	94.7	31.2	33.0	36.2	37.7	5.2	80.8	—
	Others	0.4	93.5	0.2	15.8	8.4	17.4	3.4	76.9	21.8
Acceptability of husband's extra-marital relationship	Yes	6.3	83.9	8.0	20.6	48.5	30	4.5	75.0	—
	No	93.7	85.7	91.3	25.6	51.5	27.3	94.8	75.6	100.0
Ability to refuse sex of she is not willing	Yes	4.6	90.8	90.4	26.2	79.3	31.1	—	82.5	99.7
	No	94.1	94.0	9.6	23.9	20.7	47.1	100	100.0	0.3
Total		154	459	288	112	260	130	66	356	100

* Information from the baseline survey is not presented due to change in intervention after the baseline survey.

Thus, looking at the above discussed issues of linkages between condom awareness and women's awareness on reproductive and sexual rights, no clear association is found.

Summary of findings and conclusions

- Between the baseline and endline survey, there has been a decline in STIs in four of the five CHARCA districts and that can be attributed to the increase in the capability of young women to identify the symptoms. The decline is higher among the educated and younger women.

- Except Kanpur and Guntur, young men in the remaining three districts experienced an overall decline in the symptomatic prevalence of STIs. The most frequently reported symptoms of STIs across the five districts are 'pain during urination' and 'involuntary passing of semen'.
- Utilization of public healthcare facilities among women has increased significantly in all the CHARCA districts, except in Aizawl, over the years. This result has also been supported by the increase in utilization of public healthcare providers for managing STIs in panel data. However, the utilization of public healthcare facilities for male STIs has declined.
- Perceptions of young women about the quality of care have not changed over the time period. Young women, except in Bellary, report increase in the availability of drugs in healthcare centres during the three years' period. In the case of availability of a trained doctor, young women in Kishanganj and Guntur perceive the situation to be better than the baseline. Except Aizawl, Kishanganj is the only district where healthcare components such as counselling, physical examination and follow-up advice are reported to have improved.

7

Efficacy of CHARCA Intervention

This chapter describes the impact of programmes and activities undertaken as a part of CHARCA intervention, which has been implemented for a period of almost three years with the objectives of reducing young women's vulnerability to STIs/HIV. After three years of intervention, the endline survey has been conducted to assess the expected outcomes in terms of increase in awareness, capacity building, improved reproductive and sexual health services and excellent support systems at the family and community levels. The functional efficacy of CHARCA intervention contains information pertaining to five strategies of the model adopted to reduce young women's vulnerability and translated into a programme of action through different sets of programmes and activities consistent with the local and regional situations.

The efficacy of different CHARCA intervention programmes is assessed through different scales developed after testing the reliability of statements indicating people's perception of the impact of CHARCA programmes and activities in enhancing awareness, capacity building of women, empowerment of women and improved services. Further, this chapter also aims to analyse variations in the values of scales that have been analysed by some selected socio-economic and demographic characteristics of respondents. Young women's and men's perceptions about the efficacy of CHARCA intervention are based on a set of statements canvassed to all the respondents, where their perceptions have been recorded on a five-point Likert scale ranging from 'strongly agree' to 'strongly disagree'. To ensure the negative effects of monotonous responses, the directions of the statements were changed randomly. However, in order to ensure reliability above 0.7, three of the nine factors have been removed based on factor loading. The values of the scale have been classified as *high, moderate* and *low* by selecting suitable cut-off points.

This chapter has five sections. The first section deals with the perceptions of young women and men about the efficacy of CHARCA intervention in bringing about change in the awareness level, while the perceived efficacy in empowerment of women has been presented in the second section. The third section discusses the perceived contribution of CHARCA intervention in bringing out behavioural changes in risky lifestyles of people in the project areas and perceptions of both men and women regarding improved services have been analysed in the fourth section. The last section deals with the perceived effectiveness of CHARCA programmes and activities in the overall development of women in the project areas including motivation of parents to send their girls for higher education.

Efficacy of CHARCA Intervention in enhancing awareness of STIs/HIV/AIDS

Young men's and women's perceptions about the efficacy of CHARCA intervention in enhancing awareness about STIs/HIV/AIDS have been computed based on six indicators. About 23 per cent of women and 22 per cent of men in the sample from all five districts have been excluded due to non-response. Thus, the reliability of awareness scale for women and men have been obtained as 0.72 and 0.70 respectively. The results are presented in Table 7.1 and Table 7.2.

Table 7.1 shows the variation in young women's perceptions about the efficacy of CHARCA intervention in enhancing women's awareness of STIs/HIV/AIDS issues in the five districts. Most women perceived CHARCA programmes highly important in enhancing awareness about STIs/ HIV/AIDS. In Aizawl all women perceived the CHARCA intervention as high in enhancing women's awareness, followed by Guntur (84%), Kanpur (65%), Bellary (37%) and Kishanganj (17%). Almost 95 per cent of women in Aizawl, 55 per cent in Bellary 50 per cent in Kishanganj, 34 per cent in Kanpur and 15 per cent in Guntur perceived that the CHARCA intervention has moderately enhanced women's awareness. Although less than 1 per cent women perceived about the CHARCA intervention efficacy to be low in Guntur and Kanpur districts, the proportion is much higher in other districts: 33 per cent in Kishanganj, 9 per cent in Bellary and 5 per cent in Aizawl.

Table 7.1

Percentage of women aged 13–24 perceiving efficacy of CHARCA intervention in enhancing young women's awareness of STIs/HIV/AIDS across five CHARCA districts by some selected background characteristics

Background characteristics	*Kanpur*			*Kishanganj*			*Bellary*			*Guntur*			*Aizawl*		
	High	*Moderate*	*Low*	*High*	*Moderate*	*Low*	*High*	*Moderate*	*Low*	*High*	*Moderate*	*Low*	*High*	*Moderate*	*Low*
Age															
13–16	68.9	30.3	0.8*	22.5	52.5	25	32.8	56.5	10.7	84.5	15.5	0.0	89.7	10.3	0.0
17–20	64.0	35.4	0.6*	17.2	50.0	32.8	42.7	52.4	4.9	88.5	11.5	0.0	93.1	6.9	0.0
21–24	64.2	35.8	0.0	12.5	50.0	37.5	32.7	57.0	10.3	80.5	18.9	0.6*	95.2	4.8	0.0
Education															
Illiterate	48.0	52.0	0.0	17.4	65.2	17.4	34.4	55.8	9.8	73.1	26.9	0.0	0.0	0.0	0.0
<5 years complete	61.5	38.5	0.0	15.8	57.9	15.8	15.3	72.9	11.9	81.8	18.2	0.0	50.0*	50.0*	0.0
5–7 years complete	73.9	26.1	0.0	36.1	50	36.1	40.0	52.7	7.3	84.7	14.5	0.8*	93.1	6.9*	0.0
8–9 years complete	69.3	30.7	0.0	14.3*	35.7	50.0	34.6	50.6	14.8	87.1	12.9	0.0	92.1	7.9*	0.0
10 years and above	63.3	35.7	1.0*	7.1*	32.1	60.7	46.7	51.1	2.2*	86.3	13.7	0.0	93.9	6.1	0.0
Husband's Education†															
Illiterate	50.0*	50.0*	0.0	26.3	68.4	5.3*	39.8	54	6.2	72.0	28.0	0.0	0.0	0.0	0.0
<5 years complete	0.0	0.0	0.0	29.2	37.5	33.3	15.8*	68.4	15.8*	85.7	14.3*	0.0	0.0	0.0	0.0
5–7 years complete	63.6	36.4*	0.0	13	65.2	21.7	32.6	55.8	11.6	84.2	14.7	1.1	0.0	0.0	0.0

Cont'd...

...Cont'd

8–9 years complete	54.5	45.5	0.0	7.1*	42.9	50.0	46.7	53.3	0.0	94.7	5.3*	0.0	92.9	7.1*	0.0
10 years and above	58.1	41.9	0.0	4.8*	38.1	57.1	32.3	58.5	9.2	87.8	12.2	0.0	100.0	0.0	0.0
Membership in CBOs/NGOs															
Yes	91.9	8.1	0.0	15.4*	69.2	15.4*	42.3	54.6	3.1*	86.9	12.5	0.6*	94.1	5.9	0.0
No	49.5	49.5	1.0*	0	100*	0.0	39.7	55.6	4.7	83.5	16.5	0.0	86.4	13.6	0.0
Occupation															
Homemaker	65.6	33.9	0.5*	15.1	50.6	34.3	36	54.6	9.5	85.5	14.5	0.0	92.6	7.4	0.0
Working as Labourer/family farm	53.3	46.7	0.0	50.0*	50.0*	0.0	35.4	57.7	6.9	81.5	17.3	1.2*	94.7	5.3*	0.0
Salaried/paid job	80.0*	20.0*	0.0	25.0*	75.0*	0.0	48.4	45.2	6.5*	50.0*	50.0*	0.0	100.0	0.0	0.0
Exposure to Mass Media															
Yes	65.6	34.2	0.2*	16.4	50.0	33.6	37.6	54.5	7.8	85.6	14.4	7.7*	93	7	0.0
No	63.0	33.3	3.7*	16.7	53.3	30.0	25.5	60.8	13.7	46.2	46.2	0.0	0.0	0.0	0.0
Total (N)	65.4 (282)	34.1 (147)	0.5 (2)	16.5 (29)	50.6 (89)	33 (58)	36.5 (200)	55.1 (302)	8.4 (46)	84.4 (352)	15.3 (64)	0.2 (1)	94.4 (105)	5.6 (100)	0.0 (5)

* Less than five cases.

† Based on married respondents only.

It is evident that a majority of younger women aged 13–16 perceived the intervention as highly effective except in Aizawl district where more than 95 per cent of women in older age group (aged 21–24) perceived it of high efficacy. More than 50 per cent of young women of all age groups in Bellary and Kishanganj districts and one-third in Kanpur perceived CHARCA intervention to be moderately effective.

With respect to the education of the women, clearly women who had above eight years of schooling perceived high efficacy of the intervention in almost all districts. It is worth mentioning that at least 17 per cent of the illiterate women in Kishanganj and 34 per cent women in Bellary perceived CHARCA intervention as highly efficient, which also indicates the effective reach and exposure of the intervention programmes to the uneducated women in these districts.

In addition to women's education, husband's education also indicates the influence on intervention programmes. Young women whose husbands had over five years of schooling perceived the contribution of CHARCA as highly enhancing their awareness of HIV/STIs in all districts, except in Kishanganj. Almost 40 per cent women of women whose husbands are illiterates in Bellary and 26 per cent in Kishanganj perceived the intervention as highly enhancing their awareness. In Aizawl district, all women whose husbands had education of 10 years and 94 per cent of women who had schooling of eight or more years consider the programme highly effective. Although none of the women, irrespective of their's and husband's educational levels, perceive the intervention lowly in enhancing awareness in Kanpur, Guntur and Aizawl, more than 50 per cent women who had schooling of more than eight years perceived it to be low in enhancement of their awareness.

Women members of CBOs/NGOs perceived the contribution of CHARCA as highly enhancing their awareness of HIV/STIs. Such a positive impact of intervention is shown by 94 per cent women in Aizawl, 92 per cent in Kanpur, 87 per cent in Guntur, 42 per cent in Bellary and 15 per cent in Kishanganj.

Occupation of women is another vital factor of exposure to the intervention programme. The women who are working (salaried/paid jobs) and homemakers perceived the intervention programme to be highly efficient than the women working as labourers. Among women working as homemakers, 93 per cent in Aizawl, 86 per cent in Guntur, 66 per cent in Kanpur, 36 per cent in Bellary and 15 per cent in Kishanganj perceived that the CHARCA intervention is highly enhancing women's awareness on STIs/HIV/AIDS.

Among the women who had exposure to mass media, 93 per cent in Aizawl, 86 per cent in Guntur, 66 per cent in Kanpur, 38 per cent in

Bellary and 16 per cent in Kishanganj perceived high efficacy of the intervention programme on STIs/HIV/AIDS awareness. But, the exposure to mass media did not show much variation in Kanpur and Kishanganj.

The endline survey clearly indicates that young women and men endorse the efficacy of CHARCA intervention in enhancing awareness in their communities. The efficacy is reflected among younger women, members of CBOs/NGOs, educated persons, homemakers, and those exposed to media.

Table 7.2 shows the percentage of men aged 15–29 years perceiving efficacy of CHARCA intervention in enhancing women's awareness on STIs/HIV/AIDS in the five districts. Most of the men in almost all states perceived that the intervention of CHARCA is moderately enhancing the women's awareness of STIs/HIV/AIDS. Almost 40 per cent of men in Guntur and 33 per cent men Bellary perceived high efficacy of the intervention, while it is less than 5 per cent in Aizawl and Kishanganj and less than 1 per cent in Kanpur. Men aged 20 years and above perceived the high and moderate efficacy of the intervention in all districts than their counterparts. More than one-fourth of the men in Kanpur and Kishanganj (29% and 30% respectively), 16 per cent in Bellary and 8 per cent in Aizawl perceived low efficacy of the intervention, whereas it is more than 2 per cent in Guntur district. The perception with respect to the marital status of the men reveals that the percentage of currently married men who perceived both high and moderate efficacy of the intervention is more than the never married men in all districts except Guntur. Men's occupation also reveals that the working men who perceived high and moderate efficacy of the intervention on women's awareness is slightly higher than students in almost all districts. It is worth mentioning that among the students, 33 per cent in Kanpur, 27 per cent in Kishanganj, 12 per cent in Aizawl and 6 per cent in Bellary perceived low efficacy of the intervention whereas none of the students perceived low efficacy in Guntur district. The exposure to mass media clearly shows the effect of intervention on awareness of STIs/HIV/AIDS. It is evident that among the men who had exposure to mass media had perception of high and moderate efficacy of the intervention, compared to those who did not have exposure in all districts except Bellary. It is important to note that more men with mass media exposure in Kishanganj, Guntur and Aizawl districts perceived low efficacy of the intervention than those without any such exposure.

Table 7.2

Percentage of men aged 15–29 perceiving efficacy of CHARCA intervention in enhancing young women's awareness of STIs/HIV/AIDS across five CHARCA districts by some selected background characteristics

Background characteristics	Kanpur			Kishanganj			Bellary			Guntur			Aizawl		
	High	Moderate	Low	High	Moderate	Low	High	Moderate	Low	High	Moderate	Low	High	Moderate	Low
Age															
Less than 20	0.0	74.2	25.8	4.7*	64.1	31.3	30.3	52.5	17.2	40.0	60.0	0.0	3.4*	83	13.6
20 and above	1.1*	70.0	28.9	2.6*	67.5	29.9	34.5	50.0	15.5	40.3	56.9	2.8*	3.1*	88.5	8.3
Marital Status															
Currently married	1.5	70.6	27.9	3.9*	61.8	34.2	36.0	48.3	15.7	39.7	57.3	3.9*	8.6*	80.0	11.4
Never married	0.0	72.6	27.4	2.9*	69.5	27.6	29.0	54.3	16.7	41.5	58.5	0.0	2.0*	87.2	10.7
Education															
Illiterate	50.0*	50.0*	0.0	2.6*	56.4	41.0	26.2	45.2	28.6	0.0	0.0	0.0	0.0	0.0	0.0
<5 years complete	0.0	81.8	18.2*	0.0	63.6	36.4*	25.0	57.1	17.9	28.6	71.4	0.0	100.0*	0.0	0.0
5–7 years complete	0.0	70.0	30	5.3*	57.9	36.8	18.2	56.4	25.5	47.8	49.3	2.9*	0.0	0.0	0.0
8–9 years complete	0.0	67.9	32.1	10.3*	72.4	17.2	34.3	62.9	2.9*	50	44.4	5.6	0.0	76.9	23.1*
10 years and above	0.0	74.2	25.8	0.0	75.0	25.0	46.5	47.4	6.1	38.5	60.4	1.0*	2.9	87.1	10.0
Occupation															
Student	0.0	66.7	33.3	4.7*	69.8	25.6	49.2	44.6	6.2*	36.7	63.3	0.0	2.0*	85.9	12.1

Cont'd...

...Cont'd

Working as labourer/family farm	1.1*	69.3	29.5	4.7*	55.8	39.5	30.3	52.5	17.2	43.2	54.0	2.9*	6.1*	83.7	10.2
Salaried/paid job	0.0	88.0	12.0*	0.0	80.8	19.2	16.7	53.3	30.0	30.8	69.2	0.0	2.8*	88.9	8.3*
Exposure to Mass Media															
Yes	0.7*	72.0	27.3	3.5	68.2	28.2	35.8	51.1	13.1	40.6	57.5	1.9*	3.3	85.9	10.9
No	0.0	15.0	15.0*	0.0	36.4*	63.6	14.3	50.0	35.7	0.0	100.0*	0.0	0.0	0.0	0.0
Total (N)	0.7 (1)	71.7 (109)	27.6 (42)	3.3 (6)	66.3 (120)	30.4 (55)	32.9 (104)	50.9 (161)	16.1 (51)	40.2 (86)	57.9 (124)	1.9 (4)	3.4 (6)	85.7 (158)	10.9 (200)

* Less than five cases.

'... CHARCA, Kanpur has made a significant contribution in changing the life of PLWHA in Kanpur. It is only due to the efforts made by CHARCA that a number of HIV infected persons in Kanpur came forward to disclose their identity and registered under the programme. CHARCA has taken the initiative in sending them to Lucknow for testing on a regular basis and has also helped them in getting ARTs on a regular basis. Once the number of PLWHA registered under the programme reached 33, CHARCA arranged experts for managing opportunistic infections and also organized skill development programme with a facility of drop in the centre, which was sponsored by UPSACS ...'

—FGD, project personnel, Kanpur

'... in Guntur district out of 100 persons 65 received the HIV/AIDS information from CHARCA 'kalajatha' programme. The kalajatha programme was popular in Guntur in disseminating the knowledge of HIV/AIDS and related diseases and women's vulnerability towards sexual diseases ... at village level the Anganwadi teachers and CHARCA peer educators were put on full effort. They have to go door-to-door and they to provide information about health problems apart from HIV/AIDS and also they used to give sex education ...'

—FGD, health committee workers, Guntur

To understand the success of CHARCA intervention, in-depth discussions were carried out with the general population to assess the efficacy with stakeholders like healthcare providers, programme personnel, etc. The results are similar with the survey findings. Awareness regarding the STI and HIV issues has shown a positive scenario, which is also reflected in the views expressed in the key informant interviews and focus group discussions.

Efficacy of CHARCA intervention in enhancing empowerment of women

Perceptions of CHARCA efficacy in enhancing empowerment of women have been computed based on 10 statements pertaining to programmes and activities in the project areas. In the process, one-fourth of the women and men in the sample from all five districts have been excluded due to non-response. Thus, the reliability of women's empowerment scale for women and men has been obtained as 0.78 and 0.79 respectively. Subsequently, the values of empowerment scale have been classified as *high, moderate* and *low* by selecting suitable cut-off points. The results are presented in Tables 7.3 and 7.4.

Table 7.3 shows the percentage of women aged 13–24 perceiving efficacy of the CHARCA intervention in enhancing empowerment of women across five districts. A majority of the women in almost all districts perceived moderate efficacy of the intervention in enhancing the empowerment of women in all districts. In Kanpur and Aizawl with 90 per cent of the women who perceived efficacy moderately in enhancing the empowerment is followed by 65 per cent in Bellary, 53 per cent in Guntur and 48 per cent in Kishanganj. It is worth mentioning that 47 per cent in Guntur and one-fourth in Bellary perceived that the efficacy intervention is highly enhancing, whereas the same is less than 10 per cent in Aizawl and 5 per cent in Kanpur. If we consider age, the women of age group 17–20 years perceived efficacy of the intervention as highly enhancing the women's empowerment in all districts than the other age group women. This clearly indicates that most of the women getting exposure to the intervention are of age up to 20 years. That almost one-third of the women in the age group 13–16 years in Kishanganj and one-tenth in Bellary perceived low enhancement of the intervention on empowerment of women is alarming and it is necessary for the intervention to be focused on younger women.

Only women who completed 10 or more years of schooling perceived the high enhancement of intervention in all districts except in Guntur, where the women with less than primary education level perceived the same. Among the illiterate women, 46 per cent of the women in Guntur, one-fourth in Bellary and 16 per cent in Kishanganj perceived the efficacy of intervention as highly enhancing the empowerment whereas none of the women in Kanpur and Aizawl perceived the same. Among the married women, with respect to their husband's education, women whose husband's had schooling of seven or more years perceived both high and moderate levels of enhancement than the women whose husbands were illiterate or had less than primary education.

Membership in CBOs/NGOs reveals that the members of these organizations perceive enhancement more highly than the non-members. But it is worth mentioning that in Bellary 32 per cent of the non-members perceived the efficacy of the intervention as highly enhancing. With respect to the occupation of the women, it is clearly visible that the working women as homemakers perceived the efficacy of the intervention to be of high enhancement. With regard to exposure to mass media, the women who had such exposure perceived the intervention as highly enhancing the empowerment than those who were not exposed. At the same time it is worth mentioning that the women

Table 7.3

Percentage of women aged 13–24 perceiving efficacy of CHARCA intervention in enhancing empowerment of women across five CHARCA districts by some selected background characteristics

Background characteristics	Kanpur			Kishanganj			Bellary			Guntur			Aizawl		
	High	Moderate	Low	High	Moderate	Low	High	Moderate	Low	High	Moderate	Low	High	Moderate	Low
Age															
13–16	3.7*	89	7.3	18.2	51.5	30.3	20.3	69.8	9.9	43.3	56.7	0.0	7.8	90.9	1.3*
17–20	5.6	90	4.4	15.8	49.1	35.1	30.6	62.6	6.8	50.3	49.7	0.0	12.4	86.7	0.9*
21–24	4.9	91	4.1	9.8	44.3	45.9	26.3	65.9	7.8	45.7	53.7	0.6*	7.6	92.4	0.0
Education															
Illiterate	0.0	90.9	9.1*	15.9	63.6	20.5	25.1	66.5	8.4	46.2	53.8	0.0	0.0	0.0	0.0
<5 years complete	0.0	100.0	0.0	25.0	57.1	17.9	11.7	73.3	15.0	56.1	43.9	0.0	0.0	100.0*	0.0
5–7 years complete	2.5*	92.5	5.0*	9.4*	46.9	43.8	20.7	69.4	9.9	45.2	54.0	0.8*	0.0	100.0	0.0
8–9 years complete	4.1	90.2	5.7	9.5*	28.6	61.9	26.8	64.6	8.5	41.0	59.0	0.0	12.5	86.4	1.1*
10 years and above	6.7	88.7	4.6	7.7*	26.9	65.4	37.0	60.0	3.0*	46.8	53.2	0.0	9.5	89.9	0.6*
Husband's Education†															
Illiterate	0.0	100.0	0.0	0.0	0.0	0.0	24.8	69.2	6.0	44.0	56.0	0.0	0.0	0.0	0.0
<5 years complete	0.0	0.0	0.0	10.5*	78.9	10.5*	5.3*	84.2	10.5*	57.1	42.9	0.0	0.0	0.0	0.0
5–7 years complete	8.3*	91.7	0.0	45.0	30.0	25.0	18.6	74.4	7.0*	50.0	48.9	1.1*	0.0	0.0	0.0

Cont'd...

...Cont'd

8–9 years complete	3.4*	93.1	3.4*	4.8*	81	14.2*	43.8	50.0	6.3*	57.9	42.1	0.0	0.0	100.0	0.0
10 years and above	1.5*	93.9	4.5*	0.0	25.0*	75.0	33.8	56.9	9.2	35.1	64.9	0.0	5.9*	94.1	0.0
Membership in CBOs/NGOs															
Yes	10.3	89	0.7*	18.2*	63.6	18.2*	28.9	70.1	1.0*	48	51.4	0.6*	9.1	90.5	0.4*
No	2.3*	87.9	9.8	0.0	0.0	0.0	31.9	65	3.1	47.6	52.4	0.0	11.6	86.0	2.3*
Occupation															
Homemaker	5.1	89.8	5.1	11.9	47.6	40.6	22.8	68.5	8.7	48.0	52.0	0.0	8.2	91.0	0.8*
Working as labourer/family farm	0.0	100.0*	0.0	0.0	100.0*	0.0	26.7	65.4	7.9	42.0	56.8	1.2*	16.7*	83.3	0.0
Salaried/paid job	0.0	83.3	16.7*	66.7*	33.3*	0.0	54.8	41.9	3.2*	50.0*	50.0*	0.0	30.0*	70.0	0.0
Exposure to Mass Media															
Yes	5.1	89.4	5.4	15.2	44.8	40.0	27.1	65.1	7.8	47.4	52.6	7.7*	9.5	89.4	5.4
No	0.0	100.0	0.0	7.7*	61.5	30.8	16.1	73.2	10.7	30.8*	61.5	0.0	0.0	0.0	0.0
Total (N)	4.8 (19)	90.1 (353)	5.1 (20)	13.9 (21)	47.7 (72)	38.4 (58)	25.9 (144)	65.3 (366)	5.1 (45)	46.9 (195)	52.9 (22)	0.2 (1)	9.5 (28)	89.8 (265)	0.7 (2)

* *Less than five cases.*
† *Based on married respondents only.*

with exposure to mass media also perceived low enhancement than those who had no such exposure.

Table 7.4 shows the percentage of the men aged 15–29 years perceiving efficacy of the CHARCA intervention in enhancing empowerment of women across five districts.

A majority of the men in all the districts perceived that the intervention of the CHARCA is moderately enhancing the empowerment of women. None of the men in the districts of Kanpur, Kishanganj and Aizawl perceived the intervention as highly enhancing women's empowerment, whereas 48 per cent of them in Bellary and 29 per cent in Guntur perceived so. More than one-third of the men in Aizawl district, 21 per cent in Kishanganj, 16 per cent in Kanpur, 6 per cent in Bellary and 4 per cent in Guntur districts perceived that the intervention has low enhancement in women's empowerment.

In the districts of Bellary and Guntur, the percentage of men of 20 years and above perceived that the intervention is highly enhancing the empowerment. Among the men who perceived moderate level of enhancement in the empowerment of women, it is observed that there is not much difference by their age in all districts except in Kanpur where 90 per cent of the men below 20 years and 77 per cent of 20 years and above perceived the same. The similarity can be observed by the marital status of the men in the case of those who perceived that

'... CHARCA has made significant contribution in reducing violence against women through a campaign named 'Parivartan' (means change), where women have been motivated to understand their rights in the family as well as in society and men have been motivated to understand their role in reducing violence against women at different fora. Under the campaign, CHARCA has organized special programmes for young men to make them aware of different forms of violence against women and to sensitize them to their roles and responsibilities to protect women from any form of coercion and violence ...'

—FGD functionaries, Kanpur

'... In Guntur district the CHARCA has given training at grass roots level also to adolescent girls along with the training at district level to related departments like health department, education department, ICDS, revenue department, NGOs, religious leaders, DRPs (district level resource persons), MRPs (mandal level resource persons), field supervisors, school teachers, Anganwadi teachers, health workers ...'

—FGD health committee workers, Bellary

Table 7.4

Percentage of men aged 15–29 perceiving efficacy of CHARCA intervention in enhancing empowerment of women across five CHARCA districts by some selected background characteristics

Background characteristics	*Kanpur*			*Kishanganj*			*Bellary*			*Guntur*			*Aizawl*		
	High	*Moderate*	*Low*	*High*	*Moderate*	*Low*	*High*	*Moderate*	*Low*	*High*	*Moderate*	*Low*	*High*	*Moderate*	*Low*
Age															
Less than 20	0.0	90.2	9.8	0.0	79.1	20.9	41.8	49.82	9.0	27.1	67.1	5.7*	0.0	63.6	36.4
20 and above	0.0	77.3	22.7	0.0	79.5	20.5	47.4	47.9	4.6	29.2	68.1	2.8*	0.0	67.7	32.3
Marital Status															
Currently married	0.0	77.9	22.1	0.0	72.3	27.7	43.8	48.3	7.3	30.5	67.2	2.3*	0.0	48.6	51.4
Never married	0.0	86.8	13.2	0.0	84.1	15.9	47.1	48.6	4.9	25.6	68.6	6.1	0.0	69.8	30.2
Education															
Illiterate	0.0	100.0*	0.0	0.0	71.4	28.6	40.5	47.6	11.9	0.0	0.0	0.0	0.0	0.0	0.0
<5 years complete	0.0	100.0	0.0	0.0	66.7	33.3*	42.9	50.0	7.2*	35.7	64.3	0.0	0.0	100.0*	0.0
5–7 years complete	0.0	81.0	19.0*	0.0	82.6	17.4*	38.2	54.5	3.7*	27.5	69.6	2.9*	0.0	0.0	0.0
8–9 years complete	0.0	87.1	12.9	0.0	88.0	12.0*	54.3	42.9	2.9	50.0	50.0	0.0	0.0	46.2	53.8
10 years and above	0.0	78.7	21.3	0.0	79.4	20.6	50.0	47.4	2.6*	26.0	67.7	6.3	0.0	67.1	32.9

Cont'd...

...Cont'd

Occupation															
Student	0.0	86.4	13.6	0.0	85.2	11.8*	44.6	50.8	4.6*	30.6	61.2	8.2*	0.0	67.7	32.3
Working as labourer/family farm	0.0	81.0	19.0	0.0	74.5	25.5	48.4	45.2	6.3	27.3	69.8	2.9*	0.0	59.2	40.8
Salaried/paid job	0.0	86.2	13.8*	0.0	82.4	17.6	23.3	66.7	10.0*	30.8	69.2	0.0	0.0	69.4	30.6
Exposure to Mass Media															
Yes	0.0	83.4	16.0	0.0	82.1	17.9	49.3	47.1	3.6	28.8	67.5	3.8	0.0	65.8	34.2
No	0.0	100.0*	0.0	0.0	50.0	50.0	19.0	57.1	23.8	0.0	100.0*	0.0	0.0	0.0	0.0
Total (N)	0.00 (0)	83.6 (158)	16.4 (31)	0.00 (0)	79.3 (92)	20.7 (24)	45.3 (143)	48.4 (153)	6.3 (20)	28.5 (61)	67.8 (145)	3.7 (8)	0.00 (0)	65.8 (121)	34.2 (63)

*Less than five cases.

the intervention is moderately enhancing the awareness. It is worth mentioning that the number of currently married men who perceived the efficacy of the intervention to be low is more than the men who are never married in all districts. There is not much variation among the men who perceived the efficacy of the intervention to be highly enhancing the empowerment. It is worth mentioning that even among the men who had 10 or more years of schooling, one-third in Aizawl, 21 per cent men in Kanpur and Kishanganj, 6 per cent in Guntur district and 3 per cent in Bellary perceived that the efficacy of the intervention to be not highly enhancing empowerment of the women. Among the men who perceived moderate level of enhancement, with respect to the occupation, there is not much difference that can be seen between students and salaried men. With regard to the exposure to mass media, the majority of the men who had such exposure perceived that the efficacy as moderately enhancing the empowerment of women in the districts in Kanpur, Kishanganj and Aizawl. Similarly, almost 57 per cent of the men in Bellary who had no exposure to mass media perceived the efficacy of the intervention as moderately enhancing the empowerment of the women. This is more than the 47 per cent of the men who had exposure which nullifies the impact of intervention to the exposure of mass media.

The qualitative discussions about CHARCA programme reveal its efficacy for empowering the women in terms of multi-target approach, ranging from enabling them taking their decisions to reducing gender-based violence and atrocity.

Efficacy of CHARCA intervention in reducing risk behaviours for STIs/HIV

Young women's and men's perceptions about the efficacy of CHARCA intervention in reducing risk behaviours for STIs/HIV which affects young women's vulnerability are based on a set of 10 statements canvassed to all the females aged 13–24 and males aged 15–29 included in the survey, where these have been recorded on a five-point Likert scale ranging from 'strongly agree' to 'strongly disagree'. Thus, the scale showing perceived effectiveness of CHARCA intervention in reducing risk behaviours, which in turn influences the reduced vulnerability of young women to STIs/HIV, has been computed based on six statements pertaining to the impact of CHARCA programmes and activities. In the process, 27 per cent of women and 26 per cent of men in the sample from all five districts have been excluded due to non-response. Thus, the reliability of the scale revealing perceived effectiveness of CHARCA intervention for women and men has been obtained as 0.73

and 0.80 respectively and the values of scale have been classified as *high, moderate* and *low* by selecting suitable cut-off points and the results are presented in Table 7.5 and Table 7.6.

Table 7.5 shows the percentage distribution of women aged 13–24 perceiving the efficacy of CHARCA intervention in reducing risk behaviours across five districts by some selected background characteristics. A majority of the women perceived that the efficacy of the intervention is highly enhancing in Guntur, Aizawl and Kanpur and moderately in Bellary and is low in Kishanganj. Only 1 per cent of the women in Guntur and less than 1 per cent in Kanpur and Aizawl perceived that the efficacy of the intervention has low enhancement in reducing the risk behaviours, whereas the corresponding figures for Bellary and Kishanganj are 21 per cent and 46 per cent respectively.

If we consider age, only in Kanpur, the younger women of age 13–16 years perceived the high enhancement, whereas it is the same among the other age group women in the remaining districts. Among the women of age group 17–20 years, 74 per cent in Guntur perceived high enhancement, followed by 61 per cent in Aizawl, 55 per cent in Kanpur, 21 per cent in Bellary and 18 per cent in Kishanganj. With respect to the educational level of the women, it is evident that in Kishanganj and Bellary, the illiterate women perceived high enhancement in reducing the risk behaviours, whereas in the other districts, the literates perceived the same. It is worth mentioning that among the women who had schooling of 10 years or more, almost 79 per cent in Kishanganj and 18 per cent in Bellary perceived that the efficacy of the intervention has low enhancement in reducing risk behaviour whereas the same is reported by less than 1 per cent of the women in other districts.

Among the married women, with respect to their husband's education, it is visible that a majority of the women of literate husbands reported to have perceived efficacy of the intervention as highly enhancing in reducing the risk behaviours than the women of illiterate husbands in all districts. Among the women who are the members of CBOs/NGOs, 74 per cent in Guntur, 63 per cent in Aizawl, 60 per cent in Kanpur, 23 per cent on Bellary and 15 per cent in Kishanganj perceived the efficacy as highly enhancing in reducing risk behaviours.

With respect to the occupation, it is clear that the women who are working as labourer or salaried/paid jobs perceived the efficacy of the intervention as highly enhancing in reducing the risk behaviours.

Table 7.5

Percentage of women aged 13–24 perceiving efficacy of CHARCA intervention in reducing risk behaviours across five CHARCA districts by some selected background characteristics

Background characteristics	*Kanpur*			*Kishanganj*			*Bellary*			*Guntur*			*Aizawl*		
	High	*Moderate*	*Low*	*High*	*Moderate*	*Low*	*High*	*Moderate*	*Low*	*High*	*Moderate*	*Low*	*High*	*Moderate*	*Low*
Age															
13–16	65.9	34.1	0.0	13.9	47.2	38.9	15.6	62.8	21.7	72.2	27.8	0.0	49.4	50.6	0.0
17–20	55.0	45.0	0.0	18.0	41.0	41.0	20.8	60.9	18.3	74.2	24.2	0.6*	60.9	38.3	0.9*
21–24	52.9	44.0	2.1*	12.7	32.4	54.9	15.8	61.8	22.4	68.3	28.7	3.0	67.0	33.0	0.0
Education															
Illiterate	38.5	61.5	0.0	21.3	48.9	29.8	19.4	62.4	18.2	53.8	46.2	0.0	0.0	0.0	0.0
<5 years complete	66.7	33.7*	0.0	28.1	56.3	15.6	18.6	57.6	23.7	80.3	18.2	1.5*	100.0*	0.0	0.0
5–7 years complete	68.4	31.6	0.0	5.7*	48.6	45.7	17.4	58.7	23.9	76.6	20.2	3.2*	55.2	44.8	0.0
8–9 years complete	58.7	40.4	0.9*	8.0*	12.0*	80.0	13.6	63.0	23.5	71.0	29.0	0.0	52.8	47.2	0.0
10 years and above	54.9	43.8	1.3*	6.9*	13.8*	79.3	17.3	64.7	18.0	65.9	33.3	0.7*	64.0	35.4	0.6*
Husband's Education†															
Illiterate	75.0*	25.0*	0.0	26.9	42.3	30.8	22.2	62.4	15.4	60.0	36.0	4.0*	0.0	0.0	0.0
<5 years complete	0.0	0.0	0.0	38.9	27.8	33.3	27.8	50.0	22.2	71.4	28.6	0.0	0.0	0.0	0.0
5–7 years complete	66.7	33.3*	0.0	4.8*	71.4	23.8	11.9	50.0	38.1	76.8	20.0	3.2*	0.0	0.0	0.0

Cont'd...

...Cont'd

8–9 years complete	52.2	43.5	0.0	0.0	36.4*	63.6	6.3*	87.5	6.3*	73.3	26.3	0.0	35.7	64.3	0.0
10 years and above	58.5	39.6	1.1*	0.0	14.3*	85.7	12.5	60.9	26.6	71.6	25.7	0.0	73.5	26.5	0.0
Membership in CBOs/NGOs															
Yes	60.3	39.7	0.0	15.4*	61.5	23.1*	22.9	63.5	13.5	73.9	23.9	2.3*	62.5	37.2	0.4*
No	48.5	49.2	2.3*	0.0	0.0	100.0*	19.8	64.0	16.2	70.1	29.4	0.5*	46.7	53.3	0.0
Occupation															
Homemaker	57.3	41.7	1.0*	14.5	39.0	46.5	22.8	68.5	8.7	48.0	52.0	0.0	8.2	91.0	0.8*
Working as labourer/family farm	55.6	44.4*	0.0	0.0	66.7*	33.3*	26.7	65.4	7.9	42.0	56.8	1.2	16.7*	83.3	0.0
Salaried/paid job	100.0*	0.0	0.0	33.3*	0.0	66.7*	54.8	41.9	3.2*	50.0*	50.0*	0.0	30.0*	70	0.0
Exposure to Mass Media															
Yes	56.8	42.6	0.6*	14.3	37.9	47.9	18.4	62.6	19.0	72.7	26.6	0.7*	60.1	39.6	0.3*
No	68.3	26.3	5.3*	17.9	42.9	39.3	9.4	54.7	35.8	30.8*	46.2	23.1*	0.0	0.0	0.0
Total Respondents	57.5 (185)	41.6 (134)	0.9 (3)	14.9 (25)	38.7 (65)	46.4 (78)	17.6 (96)	61.8 (338)	20.7 (113)	71.4 (297)	27.2 (113)	1.4 (6)	60.1 (179)	39.6 (118)	0.3 (1)

* Less than five cases.
† Based on married respondents only.

Except in Kanpur and Kishanganj districts, the women who were exposed to mass media had perceived high enhancement than the women who did not have such exposure. In Kanpur, 68 per cent of the women who had no exposure perceived that the intervention as highly enhancing in reducing the risk behaviours, whereas only 58 per cent who had exposure perceived the same. Almost 48 per cent of the women in Kishanganj and 19 per cent in Bellary with exposure to mass media perceived that the efficacy of the intervention as low in reducing the risk behaviours, whereas the same is reported by less than 1 per cent of the women in other districts.

Table 7.6 shows the percentage of men aged 15–29 perceiving efficacy of CHARCA intervention in reducing risk behaviours across five districts by some selected background characteristics. It is evident that a majority of the men in all districts perceived the efficacy of the intervention as highly enhancing in reducing the risk behaviours. Almost 85 per cent of the men in Guntur, 83 per cent in Kanpur, 66 per cent in Aizawl, 47 per cent in Bellary and 42 per cent in Kishanganj perceived that the efficacy of the intervention is highly enhancing in reducing the risk behaviours. However nearly 21 per cent of the men in Bellary, 12 per cent in Guntur and Kanpur and 8 per cent in Kishanganj and Aizawl perceived that the efficacy of the intervention has low enhancement in reducing the risk behaviours. Age-wise, a majority of the men below 20 years perceived the intervention to be moderately enhancing in Kanpur, Kishanganj and Aizawl districts, whereas the same is true of Bellary and Guntur districts. A similar trend can be observed in the case of men aged 20 years and above. With respect to the marital status of the men, the never married men in Kishanganj and Bellary districts perceived high enhancement, whereas the same is true of married men in Kanpur, Guntur and Aizawl districts.

The educational level of the men reveals that those who are literate and had schooling up to nine years perceived the efficacy as highly enhancing compared to the illiterates and with more than 10 years of schooling. Among the men who had more than 10 years of schooling, nearly one-fifth in Kanpur, 8 per cent in Kishanganj and Aizawl, 13 per cent in Bellary and 4 per cent in Guntur perceived that the efficacy has low enhancement in reducing the risk behaviours.

With respect to the occupation of the men, a majority in salaried/paid jobs perceived that the efficacy of the intervention as moderately enhancing in reducing the risk behaviours. It is worth as noting that among such men, 30 per cent in Bellary perceived that the intervention has low enhancement in reducing the risk behaviours

Table 7.6

Percentage of men aged 15–29 perceiving efficacy of CHARCA intervention in reducing risk behaviours across five CHARCA districts by some selected background characteristics

Background characteristics	*Kanpur*			*Kishanganj*			*Bellary*			*Guntur*			*Aizawl*		
	High	*Moderate*	*Low*	*High*	*Moderate*	*Low*	*High*	*Moderate*	*Low*	*High*	*Moderate*	*Low*	*High*	*Moderate*	*Low*
Age															
≤20	3.4*	87.9	28.6	38.3	58.3	3.3*	41.2	30.3	28.6	79.4	16.2	4.4*	27.6	63.2	9.2
>20	5.9	80.0	14.1	44.2	44.2	11.5	50.3	33.5	16.2	88.2	10.4	1.4*	24.0	68.8	7.1
Marital Status															
Currently married	8.5	76.3	15.3	36.9	46.2	16.9	44.3	31.0	24.7	87.8	10.7	1.5*	20.0	74.3	5.7*
Never married	2.4*	88.1	9.5	45.5	51.5	3.0*	50.0	33.8	16.2	81.2	15.0	3.8*	27.0	64.2	8.8*
Education															
Illiterate	50.0*	50.0*	0.0	40.0	45.7	14.3	48.8	21.4	29.8	0.0	0.0	0.0	0.0	0.0	0.0
<5 years complete	9.1*	81.8*	9.1*	30.0*	60.0	10.0*	51.9	25.9	22.2	78.6	21.4*	0.0	100.0*	0.0	0.0
5–7 years complete	5.3*	78.9	15.8*	31.4	62.9	5.7*	38.5	36.5	25.0	91.0	9.0	0.0	0.0	0.0	0.0
8–9 years complete	2.2*	95.6	2.2*	66.7	29.2	4.2*	37.1	45.7	17.1	94.4	5.6*	0.0	16.7*	75.0	8.3*
10 years and above	4.5*	77.3	18.2	41.7	50.0	8.3	50.9	35.7	13.4	82.3	13.5	4.2*	25.9	65.9	8.2

Cont'd...

...Cont'd

Occupation															
Students	2.8*	86.1	11.1*	44.7	50.0	5.3*	51.6	34.4	14.1	75.7	18.4	6.1*	25.5	66.3	8.2
Working as labourer/family farm	6.1	81.7	12.2*	37.8	51.4	10.8	48.6	29.6	21.8	88.3	10.2	1.5*	22.4	67.3	10.2
Salaried/paid job	4.2*	83.3	12.5*	46.2	46.2	7.7*	23.3	46.7	30.0	88.5	11.5	0.0	30.6	63.9	5.6
Exposure to Mass Media															
Yes	5.0	83.0	12.1	42.2	50.0	7.8	51.1	33.6	15.3	85.2	12.4	2.4	25.7	66.1	8.2
No	0.0	100.0*	0.0	40.0*	40.0*	20.0*	19.0	23.8	57.1	100.0*	0.0	0.0	0.0	0.0	0.0
Total (N)	4.9 (7)	83.2 (119)	11.9 (17)	42.1 (69)	49.4 (81)	8.5 (14)	46.8 (145)	32.3 (100)	21.0 (65)	85.4 (181)	12.3 (26)	2.4 (5)	25.7 (47)	66.1 (121)	8.2 (15)

*Less than five cases.

whereas it is around 12 per cent in Kanpur and less than 10 per cent in the remaining districts. According to the exposure to mass media, it is worth mentioning that 57 per cent of the men in Bellary and 20 per cent in Kishanganj who do not have such exposure perceived that the efficacy has low enhancement in reducing the risk behaviours, whereas none of them perceived the same in other districts.

On triangulating with qualitative findings it is found the perception and opinion at different levels regarding the CHARCA efficacy in reducing the risk behaviours among the community across the five districts lies at par with the quantitative pattern. The programme mainly targets the increase of condom awareness and use among the population, targeting alcoholism reduction among men, increasing awareness about hazards of risky sex, enabling women bargaining for condom use, promoting voluntary testing for HIV and many more sub-components.

Efficacy of CHARCA intervention in improving reproductive health services

Young women's and men's perceptions about efficacy of CHARCA intervention in improving reproductive and sexual health services are based on a set of nine statements. In order to minimize the negative effects of monotonous responses, directions of the statements were changed randomly. However, the test of reliability came out extremely high with all the nine statements and hence the scales for women and men have been computed based on all nine statements pertaining to

> '... After CHARCA many people have started coming and discussing about the safety measures of sexual activities ... the condom disposal has gone up in last few years ...'
>
> —FGD with peer educator, Bellary
>
> '... the test of HIV at different public and available outlets has increased highly ... CHARCA peer educators, while interacting with the men and women in one to one and one to many interactions, motivate the young populations ...'
>
> —KI with district resource person, Aizawl
>
> '... the women have been reaching effectively during the programme to enable themselves during sexual negotiation. At the grass roots the training is done at two levels. First, the peers are trained and then the peers organize trainings and workshops at regular intervals, which have been closely monitored ... This has affected the increasing negotiation skill among women in terms of using condom ...'
>
> —FGD with project functionaries, Kanpur

impact of CHARCA programmes and activities in improving reproductive and sexual health services in the project areas. It is worthwhile to mention that the perceived efficacy does not necessarily mean actual service utilization by the respondents but it reflects a notion which respondents carry about the programme and activities. In the process, 24 per cent of women and 21 per cent of men in the sample from all five districts have been excluded due to non-response and the reliability of scale for women and men has been obtained as 0.77 and 0.83 respectively. The response values of the service scale have been classified as *high*, *moderate* and *low* and the results are presented in Table 7.7 and Table 7.8.

Table 7.7 shows the percentage of women aged 13–24 perceiving efficacy of CHARCA intervention in improving reproductive health services across five CHARCA districts by some selected background characteristics. The efficacy of CHARCA intervention in improving the health services has been perceived as high by 81 per cent of the women in Guntur, 35 per cent in Bellary, 11 per cent in Kishanganj, 8 per cent in Kanpur and 2 per cent in Aizawl. Almost 62 per cent of the women in Kishanganj and one-third in Aizawl, 23 per cent in Kanpur and 17 per cent in Bellary perceived that the efficacy of the intervention is low in improving the reproductive health services, whereas the same is not at all perceived by any of the women in Guntur. A majority of the women in Guntur perceived high efficacy of the intervention, whereas moderate efficacy was mentioned by women in Bellary, Kishanganj and Aizawl, and the majority of the women in Kishanganj mentioned low efficacy of the intervention in improving health services. Among the younger age group women, 85 per cent of the women aged 13–16 years in Guntur perceived the high efficacy of the intervention in improving health services, where the same is mentioned by only 1 per cent of the women in Aizawl. Among the women of age group 17–20 years, a majority perceived that the efficacy of the intervention is moderately improving health services in all five districts.

With respect to the education of the women, majority of the women, irrespective of their educational level, perceived that the efficacy is moderately improving the health services in all districts. However, it is worth mentioning that among the women who had schooling more than 10 years, almost 87 per cent in Kishanganj, 34 per cent in Aizawl, 27 per cent in Kanpur and 13 per cent in Bellary district perceived the efficacy of the intervention as low in improving the health services.

Table 7.7

Percentage of women aged 13–24 perceiving efficacy of CHARCA intervention in improving reproductive health services across five CHARCA districts by some selected background characteristics

Background characteristics	*Kanpur*			*Kishanganj*			*Bellary*			*Guntur*			*Aizawl*		
	High	*Moderate*	*Low*	*High*	*Moderate*	*Low*	*High*	*Moderate*	*Low*	*High*	*Moderate*	*Low*	*High*	*Moderate*	*Low*
Age															
13–16	9.4	69.8	20.8	19.6	21.7	58.7	32.4	46.2	21.4	84.5	15.5	0.0	1.3*	60.5	38.2
17–20	6.3	72.8	20.9	6.5*	33.9	59.7	38.6	47.3	14.0	79.9	20.1	0.0	3.5*	66.7	29.8
21–24	9.0	63.9	27.0	8.7	26.1	65.2	33.5	50.3	16.2	79.9	20.1	0.0	0.0	65.4	34.6
Education															
Illiterate	5.0*	85.0	10.0*	14.0	32.0	54.0	29.2	56.0	14.9	76.9	23.1	0.0	0.0	0.0	100.0*
<5 years complete	0.0	100.0	0.0	17.6	47.1	35.3	30.0	45.0	25.0	84.8	15.2	0.0	0.0	62.1	37.9
5–7 years complete	11.6	76.8	11.6	10.3*	30.8	59.0	34.2	47.7	18.0	83.7	16.3	0.0	1.1*	67.8	31.0
8–9 years complete	3.3*	72.4	24.4	4.2*	8.3*	87.5	20.7	40.2	39.1	80.6	19.4	0.0	2.3*	64.2	33.5
10 years and above	11.2	61.5	27.3	3.3*	10.0*	86.7	43.0	43.7	13.3	77.5	22.5	0.0	1.7*	64.6	33.7
Husband's Education†															
Illiterate	0.0	100.0	0.0	15.4*	26.9	57.7	35.6	49.2	15.3	84.0	16.0	0.0	0.0	0.0	0.0
<5 years complete	0.0	0.0	0.0	20.0*	50.0	30.0	26.3	63.2	10.5*	85.7	14.3	0.0	0.0	0.0	0.0
5–7 years complete	7.7*	69.2	23.1*	9.1*	59.1	31.8	44.2	44.2	11.6	83.2	16.8	0.0	0.0	0.0	0.0

Cont'd...

...Cont'd

8–9 years complete	6.7*	73.3	20.0	0.0	16.7	83.3	31.3	62.5	6.3*	84.2	15.8	0.0	0.0	64.3	35.7
10 years and above	11.1	65.1	23.8	0.0	0.0	100.0	29.2	47.7	23.1	77.0	23.0	0.0	0.0	75.8	24.2
Membership in CBOs/NGOs															
Yes	8.0	51.1	40.9	16.7*	16.7*	66.6	30.9	64.9	4.1*	84.7	15.3	0.0	1.6*	64.7	33.7
No	10.6	73.2	16.2	0.0	0.0	100.0*	43.6	50.2	6.2	78.6	21.4	0.0	2.2*	64.4	33.3
Occupation															
Homemaker	7.9	68.4	23.7	9.6	28.7	61.7	31.5	48.6	19.8	82.7	17.3	0.0	1.9	64.5	33.6
Working as labourer/family farm	15.4*	84.6	0.0	0.0	50.0*	50.0*	37.0	50.0	13.0	75.3	24.7	0.0	0.0	73.7	26.3
Salaried/paid job	0.0	80.0*	20.0*	33.3*	0.0	66.7*	61.3	25.8	12.9*	50.0*	50.0*	0.0	0.0	50.0	50.0
Exposure to Mass Media															
Yes	8.6	67.7	23.8	10.7	28.2	61.1	36.6	47.8	15.6	81.3	18.7	0.0	1.7	64.6	33.7
No	0.0	91.7	8.3*	10.7*	25.0	64.3	21.4	48.2	30.4	69.2	30.8	0.0	0.0	0.0	0.0
Total (N)	8.0 (31)	69.2 (267)	22.8 (88)	10.7 (19)	27.7 (49)	61.6 (109)	35.1 (195)	47.8 (266)	17.1 (95)	81.0 (336)	19.0 (79)	0.00 (0)	1.7 (5)	64.6 (190)	33.7 (99)

* Less than five cases.

† Based on married respondents only.

Seventy-eight per cent young women in Guntur whose husbands had schooling of more than 10 years perceived highly of CHARCA intervention to improve reproductive health services, followed by 29 per cent in Bellary and 11 per cent in Kanpur, but by only 3 per cent in Kishanganj and 2 per cent in Aizawl. Also, contrary to expectation, in four districts majority of women who are not members of CBOs/NGOs perceived as high CHARCA intervention to improve health services. It is worth mentioning that there are substantial proportions of women who are members of CBOs/NGOs in most districts who perceived lowly the CHARCA intervention. The proportions are 67 per cent in Kishanganj, 41 per cent in Kanpur and 34 per cent in Aizawl. With respect to the occupation of the women, it is evident that among the women working as homemakers, a majority perceived the efficacy of the intervention to be moderate in Kanpur, Bellary and Aizawl whereas the women doing service/paid jobs perceived the same in Guntur and Kanpur. Among the women who had exposure to mass media, 81 per cent in Guntur, 37 per cent in Bellary, 11 per cent in Kishanganj, 8 per cent in Kanpur and less than 2 per cent in Aizawl perceived that the efficacy of the intervention is high in providing the reproductive health services.

Table 7.8 shows the percentage of men aged 15–29 perceiving efficacy of CHARCA intervention in improving reproductive health services across five CHARCA districts by some selected background characteristics. It is evident that a majority of the men in all districts perceived the efficacy of the intervention to be moderate in improving health services in the districts of Kanpur, Kishanganj and Aizawl. Almost 81 per cent of the men in Guntur and 68 per cent in Bellary perceived the efficacy high in improving the reproductive health services. However, nearly 14 per cent in Aizawl and Kanpur each, 5 per cent in Bellary and 2 per cent in Kishanganj perceived the efficacy as low.

A majority of the men aged below 20 years perceived the intervention moderately in Kanpur, Kishanganj and Aizawl districts, and high in Bellary and Guntur districts. A similar trend can be observed in the case of men aged 20 years and above. With respect to the marital status of the men, the never married men in Bellary district perceived efficacy higher than the younger men, whereas the same is true of married men in Kanpur, Guntur and Aizawl districts.

The educational level of the men reveals that the men who are literate and had schooling up to nine years perceived the efficacy as high in providing the reproductive health services, compared to the illiterates and those who had schooling more than 10 years. Among the men who had schooling more than 10 years, nearly 19 per cent in

Table 7.8

Percentage of men aged 15–29 perceiving efficacy of CHARCA intervention in improving reproductive health services across five CHARCA districts by some selected background characteristics

Background characteristics	*Kanpur*			*Kishanganj*			*Bellary*			*Guntur*			*Aizawl*		
	High	*Moderate*	*Low*	*High*	*Moderate*	*Low*	*High*	*Moderate*	*Low*	*High*	*Moderate*	*Low*	*High*	*Moderate*	*Low*
Age															
Less than 20	1.1*	91.1	7.8	0.0	96.7	3.3*	63.1	30.3	6.6	75.7	24.3	0.0	6.8	75.0	18.2
20 and above	9.8	71.6	18.6	6.9*	98.2	0.9*	70.6	25.3	4.8	83.3	16.7	0.0	7.3	83.3	9.4
Marital Status															
Currently married	9.3	69.3	21.3	0.0	98.7	1.3*	65.7	28.1	6.2	84.0	16.0	0.0	2.9*	80.0*	17.1
Never married	3.4*	88.0	8.5	1.1*	96.8	2.1*	70.3	26.1	3.6	75.6	24.4	0.0	8.1	79.2	12.8
Education															
Illiterate	0.0	100.0*	0.0	0.0	94.9	5.1*	16.9	28.6	9.5	0.0	0.0	0.0	0.0	0.0	0.0
<5 years complete	25.0*	66.7*	8.3*	0.0	100.0	0.0	64.3	25.0	10.7*	78.6	21.4	0.0	0.0	100.0*	0.0
5–7 years complete	9.1*	72.7*	18.2*	0.0	100.0	0.0	60.0	30.9	9.1	76.8	23.2	0.0	0.0	0.0	0.0
8–9 years complete	3.1*	90.8	6.2*	0.0	100.0	0.0	74.3	25.7	0.0	88.9	11.1*	0.0	0.0	69.2	30.8*
10 years and above	4.4*	76.9	18.7	1.9*	96.2	1.9*	74.6	25.4	0.0	82.3	17.7	0.0	7.6	80.0	12.4

Cont'd...

...Cont'd

Occupation															
Students	1.8*	82.5	15.8	2.8*	97.2	0.0	70.8	29.2	0.0	79.6	20.4	0.0	5.1	82.8	12.1
Working as labourer/family farm	7.8	79.4	12.7	0.0	96.3	3.7*	70.1	24.0	5.9	82.0	18.0	0.0	8.2*	67.3	24.5
Salaried/paid job	6.5*	80.6	12.9*	0.0	100.0	0.0	43.3	46.7	10.0	76.9	23.1	0.0	11.1*	86.1	2.8*
Exposure to Mass Media															
Yes	5.8	80.5	13.7	0.6*	98.1	1.3*	71.5	26.3	2.2	81.1	18.9	0.0	7.1	79.3	13.6
No	0.0	100.0*	0.0	0.0	90.9	9.1*	42.9	33.3	23.8	50.0*	50.0*	0.0	0.0	0.0	0.0
Total (N)	5.7 (11)	80.7 (155)	13.5 (26)	0.6 (1)	97.1 (167)	1.8 (3)	67.7 (214)	27.2 (86)	5.1 (16)	80.8 (173)	19.2 (41)	0.00 (0)	7.1 (13)	79.3 (146)	13.6 (25)

* Less than five cases.

Kanpur, 8 per cent in Aizawl and 2 per cent in Kishanganj perceived the efficacy to be low in providing reproductive health services.

With regard to the occupation of the men, a majority of the students and the men pursuing salaried/paid jobs perceived that the efficacy of the intervention is moderate in providing reproductive health services. It is worth noting that among the men who are working as labourers, 8 per cent in Kanpur, 70 per cent in Bellary, 82 per cent in Guntur perceived that the efficacy of the intervention is high in providing reproductive health services. Contrarily, 14 per cent in Kanpur and Aizawl each, who had exposure to mass media, had perceived that the efficacy of the intervention is low in providing the reproductive health services.

Similarly, the qualitative findings regarding CHARCA programme impact in improving reproductive health services reveal the success story of the programme. The programme has not only strengthened the services by sensitizing the people, but also made women aware as well as enables them to access the public healthcare facilities.

Efficacy of CHARCA intervention in motivating parents to send girls for higher education and overall development of women

Table 7.9 shows the percentage of women aged 13–24 perceiving efficacy of CHARCA intervention in motivating parents to send girls for higher education across five CHARCA districts by some selected background characteristics. A majority of the women perceived that the efficacy of the intervention in motivating girls for higher education

> '... CHARCA has benefited in improving the healthcare behaviour of young women and men by enabling them to access the public healthcare system ... the peer educators not only provide awareness and motivation to go for correct treatment at a right time but they also follow up the young women about the regular touch ups ...'
>
> —Interview with DRP, Guntur
>
> '... CHARCA has empowered the young women in terms of educating them about the right way of healthcare system which has increased the number of women looking towards public healthcare providers at the time of need and further in terms of advocacy of getting the right treatment as a rights-based approach ... our functionaries also monitor closely the delivering quality of services to the young women at different levels ...'
>
> —Interview with DRP, Bellary

is high in all the districts. It is worth mentioning that none of the women in Guntur perceived the efficacy of the intervention to be low, whereas 27 is 8 per cent in Kanpur, 13 per cent in Kishanganj, 3 per cent in Bellary and less than 1 per cent in Aizawl.

If we consider age, while in Aizawl only the younger women aged 13–16 years perceived the efficacy of the intervention in motivating parents to send their girls for higher education as high, the same is true of the women in the age group 17–20 years. Among the women of age group 17–20 years, 97 per cent in Guntur perceived the efficacy as high, followed by 78 per cent in Aizawl, 77 per cent in Kanpur, 71 per cent in Bellary and 47 per cent in Kishanganj. With respect to the educational level of the women, it is evident that the women who had schooling up to secondary level education perceived the intervention high in providing higher education to girls. It is worth mentioning that among the women who had 10 year or more schooling, almost 97 per cent in Guntur, 79 in Aizawl and 75 per cent in Bellary perceived that the efficacy of the intervention is high in providing higher education to girls. Among the married women, with respect to their husband's education, it is clear that a majority of the women of literate husbands are reported to have also perceived that efficacy of the intervention as high in providing the higher education to girls than the women of illiterate husbands in all districts. Among the women who are not the members of CBOs/NGOs, 96 per cent in Guntur, 89 per cent in Aizawl, 70 per cent in Kanpur, 77 per cent on Bellary and 68 per cent in Kishanganj perceived the efficacy as high in providing higher education to girls.

With respect to the occupation of the women, it is clear that the women who are working as labourers or doing salaried/paid jobs perceived the efficacy of the intervention as high in providing the higher education to girls. According to the exposure of mass media, women who had such exposure perceived high than those not exposed. In Guntur district 77 per cent of the women with no exposure perceived the intervention to be high in providing the higher education to girls, followed by 72 per cent in Kanpur, 59 in Bellary 40 per cent in Kishanganj. Around 11 per cent of the women in Kishanganj district reported that they perceived the efficacy as low in providing the higher education to girls.

Table 7.10 shows the percentage of men aged 15–29 perceiving efficacy of CHARCA intervention in improving the parents' attitude towards education of girls across five CHARCA districts by some selected background characteristics. It is evident that a majority of the

Table 7.9

Percentage of women aged 13–24 perceiving efficacy of CHARCA intervention in motivating parents to send girls for higher education across five CHARCA districts by some selected background characteristics

Background characteristics	Kanpur			Kishanganj			Bellary			Guntur			Aizawl		
	High	Moderate	Low	High	Moderate	Low	High	Moderate	Low	High	Moderate	Low	High	Moderate	Low
Age															
13–16	75.9	24.1	0.0	44.4	43.2	12.3	67.0	30.8	2.2*	95.9	4.1*	0.0	84.8	15.2	0.0
17–20	76.5	21.6	2.0	47.4	39.5	13.2	71.0	25.6	3.4	96.8	3.2	0.0	77.6	21.6	0.0
21–24	62.7	29.7	7.6	48.8	38.0	13.2	67.1	30.5	2.4*	93.9	6.1	0.0	83.0	17.0	0.0
Education															
Illiterate	53.2	36.2	10.6	51.6	39.8	8.6	65.5	31.0	3.6	96.2	3.8*	0.0	0.0	0.0	0.0
<5 years complete	75.0	25.0	0.0	58.5	33.8	7.7	60.0	35.0	5.0*	97.0	3.0*	0.0	100.0*	0.0	0.0
5–7 years complete	79.7	20.3	0.0	44.9	40.6	14.5	71.2	27.0	1.8*	95.25	4.8	0.0	79.3	20.7	0.0
8–9 years complete	74.0	25.0	1.0*	38.0	40.0	22.0	65.9	30.5	3.7*	90.3	9.7	0.0	86.7	13.3	0.0
10 years and above	72.1	23.8	4.0	36.2	46.8	17.0	75.6	23.7	0.7*	97.1	2.9*	0.0	78.9	20.6	0.6*
Husband's Education†															
Illiterate	50.0	41.7	8.3*	46.7	51.1	2.2*	67.8	28.0	4.2	92.0	8.0*	0.0	0.0	0.0	0.0
<5 years complete	66.7*	0.0	33.3*	63.6	27.3	9.1*	73.7	26.3	0.0	100.0	0.0	0.0	0.0	0.0	0.0
5–7 years complete	66.7	22.2*	11.1*	60.5	31.6	7.9*	62.8	27.9	9.3*	93.7	6.3	0.0	0.0	0.0	0.0

Cont'd...

...Cont'd

8–9 years complete	56.0	36.0	80*	39.1	39.1	21.7	62.5	32.5	0.0	94.7	5.3*	0.0	78.6	21.4*	0.4*
10 years and above	69.9	22.3	7.8	34.5	34.5	31.0	69.2	29.2	1.5*	95.9	4.1*	0.0	85.3	14.7	0.0
Membership in CBOs/NGOs															
Yes	67.4	32.6	0.0	42.1	47.4	10.5*	80.4	19.6	0.0	95.5	4.5	0.0	30.1	19.5	0.0
No	71.3	25.6	3.0	66.7*	33.3*	0.0	76.7	22.6	0.8*	95.3	4.7	0.0	88.9	11.1	0.0
Occupation															
Homemaker	71.4	25.6	3.0	47.7	39.1	13.2	68.5	28.2	3.3	96.37	3.3	0.0	81.3	18.4	0.4*
Working as labourer/family farm	88.0	12.0*	0.0	28.6*	57.1*	14.3*	67.2	30.7	2.1*	90.1	9.9	0.0	89.5	10.5*	0.0
Salaried/paid job	85.7	0.0	14.3*	62.5	25.0*	12.5*	77.4	22.6	0.0	100.0*	0.0	0.0	70.0	30.0*	0.0
Exposure to Mass Media															
Yes	72.2	25.3	2.4	48.9	39.8	11.4	69.6	28.2	2.2	96.0	4.0	0.0	81.4	18.3	0.3*
No	72.1	18.2	9.1	40.0	40.0	20.0	58.9	33.9	7.1*	76.9	23.1*	0.0	0.0	0.0	0.0
Total (N)	62.7 (116)	29.7 (55)	7.6 (14)	47.2 (153)	39.8 (129)	13.0 (42)	68.5 (38)	28.8 (160)	2.7 (15)	95.4 (398)	4.6 (19)	0.00 (0)	81.4 (245)	18.3 (55)	0.3 (1)

* Less than five cases.

† Based on married respondents only.

men in all districts perceived that the efficacy of the intervention is low in Guntur, Bellary, Kishanganj and Aizawl districts, whereas it is high in Kanpur district. Almost 95 per cent of the men in Guntur, 94 per cent in Bellary, 61 per cent in Kishanganj, 48 per cent in Aizawl and 47 per cent in Kanpur perceived efficacy of the intervention as low in providing higher education for girls.

The age distribution indicates that a majority of men aged below 20 years perceived as low the intervention in providing higher education to girls in Kishanganj (60%), Bellary (88%) and Aizawl (83%). A similar trend is observed in the case of men aged 20 years and above. With respect to the marital status of the men, the never married men in Bellary district perceived that the efficacy of the intervention as high in providing higher education to girls than the younger men, whereas the same is true of married men in Kanpur, Guntur and Aizawl districts.

The educational level of the men reveals that the men who are literate and had schooling up to nine years perceived the efficacy of the intervention in providing the higher education to girls as high compared to the illiterates. Among the men who had schooling of more than 10 years, nearly 47 per cent in Kanpur, 60 per cent in Kishanganj, 90 per cent in Bellary and 95 in Guntur perceived the efficacy of the intervention as low in providing higher education to girls.

So far as the occupation of men is concerned a majority of students and men pursuing salaried/paid jobs perceived the efficacy of the intervention as low in providing higher education to girls. According to the exposure to mass media, it is worth mentioning that 95 per cent in Guntur, 94 per cent in Bellary, 47 per cent in Kanpur, 61 per cent in Kishanganj and 48 per cent in Aizawl, who had exposure to mass media, perceived that the efficacy of the intervention to be low in providing higher education to girls.

Table 7.11 shows the percentage of women aged 13–24 perceiving efficacy of CHARCA intervention in benefiting the younger women across five CHARCA districts by some selected background characteristics. All women in Aizawl perceived that the efficacy of the intervention is high in benefiting the younger women, followed by 98 per cent in Guntur, 89 per cent in Kanpur, 86 per cent in Bellary and 76 per cent in Kishanganj. Only 5 per cent women in Kanpur perceived the efficacy as low in benefiting the younger women, whereas the same is less than 1 per cent in Kishanganj and Bellary and none of the women perceived it as low in Guntur and Aizawl.

Table 7.10

Percentage of men aged 15–29 perceiving efficacy of CHARCA intervention in improving the parents' attitude in education of girls across five CHARCA districts by some selected background characteristics

Background characteristics	Kanpur			Kishanganj			Bellary			Guntur			Aizawl		
	High	Moderate	Low	High	Moderate	Low	High	Moderate	Low	High	Moderate	Low	High	Moderate	Low
Age															
Less than 20	3.6	55.5	40.9	3.3*	36.7	60.0	6.6	5.7	87.7	0.0	5.7*	94.3	10.2	36.4	83.4
20 and above	4.7	42.6	42.7	7.6	31.0	61.4	3.6	5.2	91.2	0.0	4.2	95.8	13.5	42.7	43.7
Marital Status															
Currently married	7.5	43.9	48.6	10.3	36.1	53.6	6.2	5.6	88.2	0.0	4.6	95.4	14.3	48.6	37.1
Never married	2.2*	51.7	46.1	2.9*	31.2	65.9	2.9*	5.1	92.0	0.0	4.9*	95.1	11.4	37.6	51.0
Education															
Illiterate	0.0	50.0*	50.0*	7.7*	26.9	65.4	9.5	8.3	82.1	0.0	0.0	0.0	0.0	0.0	0.0
<5 years complete	0.0	42.1	57.9	18.8*	18.8*	62.5	7.1*	7.1*	85.7	0.0	7.1*	92.9	0.0	0.0	100.0*
5–7 years complete	3.1*	53.1	43.8	3.9*	43.1	52.9	9.1	7.3*	83.6	0.0	4.3*	95.7	0.0	0.0	0.0
8–9 years complete	2.3*	52.3	45.3	2.6	28.9	68.4	0.0	8.6*	91.4	0.0	11.1*	88.9	15.9*	30.8*	53.8
10 years and above	6.2	46.6	47.3	5.1*	35.9	59.0	0.0	0.9*	99.1	0.0	3.1*	96.3	11.8	40.6	47.6

Cont'd...

...Cont'd

Occupation															
Students	5.3	52.6	42.1	3.4*	36.2	60.3	0.0	4.6*	95.4	0.0	4.1*	95.9*	11.1	38.4	0.0
Working as labourer/family farm	4.0	49.3	46.7	8.0	32.1	59.8	0.0	5.0	89.6	0.0	5.8	95.2	12.2	34.7	0.0
Salaried/paid job	2.9*	34.3	62.9	4.6*	32.3	63.1	10.0*	10.0*	80.0	0.0	0.0	100.0	13.9	50.0	50.5
Exposure to Mass Media															
Yes	4.2	48.4*	47.3	5.9	32.9	61.3	1.3*	4.4	94.2	0.0	4.7	95.3	12.0	39.7	48.3
No	0.0	100.0*	0.0	7.7*	38.5	53.8	26.2	11.9	61.9	0.0	0.0	100.0*	0.0	0.0	0.0
Total (N)	4.2 (12)	48.8 (139)	47.0 (134)	6.0 (14)	33.2 (78)	60.9 (143)	4.7 (15)	5.4 (17)	89.9 (284)	0.00 (0)	4.7 (10)	95.3 (204)	12.0 (22)	39.7 (73)	48.4 (89)

*Less than five cases.

The older women aged 21–24 years in all districts perceived the efficacy of the intervention as high in benefiting the younger women compared to the women of other age groups. Nearly 28 per cent of women aged 13–16 in Kanpur, 22 per cent of women aged 17–20 and 19 per cent of women aged 20 years and above perceived the efficacy of the intervention as low in benefiting the younger women. With respect to the educational level of the women, there is not much variation in perceiving the efficacy of the intervention as highly benefiting the younger women in Aizawl district with marginal differentials in other districts. However, only in Kishanganj and Bellary districts, a considerable proportion of women reported that they perceived the efficacy of the intervention as moderate in benefiting the younger women, irrespective of their background characteristics.

It is worth mentioning that exposure to mass media among women does not lead to much variation in perceiving the efficacy of the intervention in Kishanganj. However, among the members of CBOs/NGOs, a majority perceived that the efficacy is high in Kanpur and Kishanganj and the same is low in Bellary.

There is no variation observed with respect to the membership in the CBOs/NGOs in case of Guntur and Aizawl districts. The similarity can be observed with respect to their occupation where the women who are working as homemakers had reported the efficacy of the intervention as high in benefiting the younger women in Kanpur and Kishanganj and not much variation in Guntur compared to their counterparts.

Table 7.12 shows the percentage of men aged 15–29 perceiving efficacy of CHARCA intervention in benefiting the younger women across five CHARCA districts by some selected background characteristics. It is evident that majority of the men in all districts perceived the efficacy of the intervention as low in all districts. None of the men in Kanpur and Guntur districts mentioned high as their perception on efficacy of the intervention whereas it is less than 5 per cent in the remaining districts. More than one-fourth of the men in Kishanganj and one-fifth in Kanpur, besides 18 per cent in Aizawl, 5 per cent in Bellary and 3 per cent in Guntur, perceived the efficacy of the intervention in benefiting the younger women as moderate. With respect to the educational level of the men, it is clearly visible that the men who had fewer years of schooling had perceived low efficacy of the intervention in benefiting the younger women. The similarity can also be observed

Table 7.11

Percentage of women aged 13–24 perceiving efficacy of CHARCA intervention in benefiting the younger women across five CHARCA districts by some selected background characteristics

Background characteristics	*Kanpur*			*Kishanganj*			*Bellary*			*Guntur*			*Aizawl*		
	High	*Moderate*	*Low*	*High*	*Moderate*	*Low*	*High*	*Moderate*	*Low*	*High*	*Moderate*	*Low*	*High*	*Moderate*	*Low*
Age															
13–16	89.0	6.3	4.7	70.4	28.4	1.2*	85.7	13.7	0.5*	97.9	2.1*	0.0	100.0	0.0	0.0
17–20	87.5	5.5	7.1	75.7	22.6	1.7*	85.0	14.0	1.0*	98.1	1.9*	0.0	100.0	0.0	0.0
21–24	91.9	4.9	3.2	80.6	19.4	0.0	86.2	12.6	1.2*	98.8	1.2*	0.0	100.0	0.0	0.0
Education															
Illiterate	89.4	2.1*	8.5*	87.1	12.9	0.0	86.3	12.5	1.2*	100.0	0.0	0.0	100.0	0.0	0.0
<5 years complete	80.0	10.0*	10.0*	83.1	16.9	0.0	80.0	18.3	1.7*	98.5	1.5*	0.0	100.0	0.0	0.0
5–7 years complete	91.9	4.1*	4.1*	75.7	24.3	0.0	82.0	17.1	0.9*	98.4	1.6*	0.0	100.0	0.0	0.0
8–9 years complete	88.5	6.3	5.2	62.0	34.0	4.0*	84.1	14.6*	1.2*	98.4	1.6*	0.0	100.0	0.0	0.0
10 years and above	89.6	5.7	4.7	61.7	36.2	2.1*	91.1	8.9	0.0	97.8	2.2	0.0	100.0	0.0	0.0
Husband's Education†															
Illiterate	91.7	0.0	8.3*	91.1	8.9*	0.0	84.7	14.4	0.8*	100.0	0.0	0.0	0.0	0.0	0.0
<5 years complete	100.0*	0.0	0.0	87.9	12.1*	0.0	84.2	15.8*	0.0	100.0	0.0	0.0	0.0	0.0	0.0
5–7 years complete	94.4	0.0	5.6*	76.3	23.7	0.0	79.1	20.9	0.0	98.9	1.1*	0.0	0.0	0.0	0.0

Cont'd...

...Cont'd

8–9 years complete	86.0	10.0	4.0*	82.6	17.4*	0.0	87.5	12.5*	0.0	100.0	0.0	0.0	100.0	0.0	0.0
10 years and above	93.2	3.9*	2.9*	60.0	40.0	0.0	86.2	13.8	0.0	98.6	1.4*	0.0	100.0	0.0	0.0
Membership in CBOs/NGOs															
Yes	95.7	2.8*	1.4*	84.2	15.8*	0.0	89.7	9.3	1.0*	98.3	1.7*	0.0	100.0	0.0	0.0
No	86.0	7.9	6.1	66.7*	33.3*	0.0	93.4	6.6	0.0	98.6	1.4*	0.0	100.0	0.0	0.0
Occupation															
Homemaker	89.8	5.7	4.5	76.7	22.3	1.0*	84.1	15.3	0.6*	98.5	1.5	0.0	100.0	0.0	0.0
Working as labourer/family farm	80.0	0.0	20.0	71.4	28.6*	0.0	88.0	10.9	1.0*	97.5	2.5*	0.0	100.0	0.0	0.0
Salaried/paid job	71.4	14.3*	14.3*	62.5	37.5*	0.0	87.1	9.7	3.2*	100.0	0.0	0.0	100.0	0.0	0.0
Exposure to Mass Media															
Yes	88.9	5.9	5.2	76.6	22.3	1.1*	87.6	11.8	0.6*	98.5	1.5	0.0	100.0	0.0	0.0
No	92.7	1.8*	5.5	75.0	25.0	0.0	67.9	28.6	3.6	92.3	7.7	0.0	0.0	0.0	0.0
Total	89.2	5.5	5.2	76.3	22.8	0.9	85.6	13.5	0.9	98.3	1.7	0.0	100.0	0.00	0.00
Respondents	(563)	(35)	(33)	(348)	(74)	(3)	(476)	(75)	(5)	(410)	(7)	(0)	(301)	(0)	(0)

* Less than five cases.

† Based on married respondents only.

with regard to the exposure of mass media, where the men who did not have exposure had perceived low efficacy in benefiting the younger women.

The multi-faceted approach of CHARCA programmes not only targeted the young women but also other stakeholders of community and familial life set-up for a sound support system and a conducive enabling environment. The efficacy of sensitizing and motivating the behaviour of the parents and other stakeholders gets reflected in the qualitative findings from Kanpur district which is getting echoed throughout the CHARCA districts.

'... an illiterate woman from Singhpur village, aged 45, working as labourer to earn day-to-day livelihood for herself and three children, was so impressed with the messages on education and rights of women that she came through CHARCA programmes that she decided to continue education of her daughter even in spite of poor economic condition. Her daughter has passed high school in 2005–06 and currently attending college at Kanpur from where she commutes every day ...'

—Interview with peer educator, Kanpur

'... A girl in a remote village of Kanpur rural, educated up to 10th standard but attended Kishori training programme 5–6 times in her own village as well as by visiting neighbouring villages along with her other female friends, was so impressed with the messages about women's rights that she declined to marry an older groom. In fact, she belongs to a low socio-economic family where parents did not have capacity to pay heavy cash or kind as dowry. She discontinued her education after passing 10th standard but was in a continuous touch of the women's resource centres working in her village as well as in the neighbouring villages (where one of her friends was actively involved in CHARCA programmes and activities). After a couple of years of efforts in getting a suitable match for the girl, parents could manage a groom, who was 15 years older than her. On the marriage day, when groom side came to her village to marry her, somehow she got this message that her would-be husband is a widower and having one son from his first wife. She discussed with her other female friends and declined to marry that gentleman. Within no time even other girls and women from the village came forward to support her, which was further supported even by male members of the village ...'

—FGD project functionaries, Kanpur

Table 7.12

Percentage of men aged 15–29 perceiving efficacy of CHARCA intervention in benefiting the younger women across five CHARCA districts by some selected background characteristics

Background characteristics	Kanpur			Kishanganj			Bellary			Guntur			Aizawl		
	High	Moderate	Low	High	Moderate	Low	High	Moderate	Low	High	Moderate	Low	High	Moderate	Low
Age															
≤20	0.0	21.7	78.3	1.1*	24.2	74.7	5.7	5.7	88.5	0.0	5.7	0.0	2.3*	23.9	73.9
>20	0.7	31.3	68.0	6.0	27.8	66.8	2.6	5.2	92.3	0.0	2.1*	97.9	3.1*	12.5	84.4
Marital Status															
Currently married	0.9*	39.4	59.6	8.8	32.4	58.8	4.5	5.1	90.4	0.0	2.3*	97.7	0.0	28.6	71.4
Never married	0.0	19.0	81.0	0.7*	22.1	77.1	2.9*	5.8	91.3	0.0	4.9*	95.1	3.4	15.4	81.2
Education															
Illiterate	0.0	100.0*	0.0	1.9*	26.9	71.2	8.3	6.0	85.7	0.0	0.0	0.0	0.0	0.0	0.0
<5 years complete	0.0	15.8*	84.2	11.8*	17.6*	70.6	3.6*	14.3	82.1	0.0	7.1*	92.9	0.0	0.0	100.0*
5–7 years complete	0.0	31.3	68.8	0.0	40.4	59.6	7.3*	7.3*	85.5	0.0	2.9*	97.1	0.0	0.0	0.0
8–9 years complete	0.0	30.2	69.8	5.0*	20.0	75.0	0.0	2.9	97.1	0.0	5.6*	94.4	0.0	38.5	61.5
10 years and above	0.7*	24.2	75.2	6.2	22.2	71.6	0.0	2.6	97.4	0.0	2.1*	97.9	2.9	16.5	80.6

Cont'd...

...Cont'd

Occupation															
Students	0.0	21.9	78.1	1.7*	20.7	77.6	0.0	3.1*	96.9	0.0	4.1*	95.9	3.0*	18.2	78.8
Working as labourer/family farm	0.7	26.3	73.0	4.4	32.5	63.2	4.5	5.9	89.6	0.0	3.6	96.4	4.1*	20.4	75.5
Salaried/paid job	0.0	42.9	57.1	5.7*	21.4	72.9	6.7*	6.7*	86.7	0.0	0.0	100.0	0.0	13.9	86.1
Exposure to Mass Media															
Yes	0.3*	26.2	73.4	4.4	26.2	69.4	1.5*	5.5	93.1	0.0	3.3	96.7	2.7	17.9	79.3
No	0.0	100.0*	0.0	0.0	30.8*	69.2	19.0	4.8*	76.2	0.0	0.0	100.0	0.0	0.0	0.0
Total (N)	0.0 (0)	21.7 (30)	78.3 (108)	4.1 (10)	26.4 (64)	69.4 (168)	3.8 (12)	5.4 (17)	90.8 (287)	0.00 (0)	3.3 (7)	96.7 (207)	2.7 (5)	17.9 (33)	79.3 (146)

* Less than five cases.

Summary of findings and conclusions

- Most young women in all the districts under survey perceive that the intervention of CHARCA has highly enhanced awareness about STIs/HIV/AIDS among people in the project areas. Since assessment of efficacy is based on perceptions, there is a clear difference in the perceived efficacy by education. Women having more than eight years of schooling are more likely to perceive high efficacy of the intervention programme in almost all districts. Women who had exposure to mass media described CHARCA programmes on STIs/HIV/AIDS as highly effective. However, exposure to mass media did not have much impact in Kanpur and Kishanganj.
- Members of CBOs/NGOs perceived the intervention to have high efficacy than non-members. But, in Bellary district, there is no significant difference in the opinions about the perceived efficacy of the programmes between members and non-members. With respect to occupation, most young women who are homemakers considered highly the efficacy of the intervention. Also, women working as labourers or doing salaried/paid jobs perceived highly the efficacy of the intervention in reducing risk behaviours.
- A majority of the men in all the five districts perceived the CHARCA intervention to be moderately efficient in empowering women. None of the men in Kanpur, Kishanganj and Aizawl perceived the intervention to be highly effective in empowering women. Married women who have literate husbands considered CHARCA intervention as highly effective in reducing the risky behaviour as women who have illiterate husbands.
- Perceptions regarding the efficacy of CHARCA intervention on different issues have been varying. For instance, a majority of respondents considered that CHARCA intervention has been effective on matters related to reducing risk behaviour (as in Aizawl, Guntur and Kishanganj), beneficial to women and in encouraging young women for higher education.
- Most responses also suggest that the intervention has not been very much effective in improving services and in empowering women.

8

Summary and Conclusions

The recent evidence about the HIV infection indicate an increasing female-male ratio and its concentration among youth, particularly adolescents. The current scenario primarily entails a concerted effort for prevention and control, which should be designed keeping in view the risks associated with the vulnerability of young women in the rural areas of the country. In view of the risk behaviour dimensions of adolescents and young adults (below 25 years), the efforts of CHARCA (Coordinated HIV/AIDS response through Capacity-Building and Awareness) to reduce the vulnerability of young women aged 13–24 from HIV infection in five selected districts in India are timely and need-based.

The CHARCA project is a coordinated initiative of the various UN agencies that aims to empower women to protect themselves against STIs/HIV using a rights-based holistic approach. The project recognizes the fact that women, given their overall low and marginal status in society, are at greater risk of acquiring HIV. The essential elements of the CHARCA programme are:

- to provide information related to sexually transmitted infections (STIs) and rights issues;
- to improve accessibility of quality services;
- to build capacity and a supporting network by providing a conducive environment that will empower women to protect themselves against STIs/HIV; and
- to assert their rights effectively.

As part of the CHARCA evaluation plan, the International Institute for Population Sciences (IIPS), Mumbai, at the request of United Nations Development Programme, undertook the task of conducting a baseline survey in five districts.* The primary objective of the CHARCA baseline survey was to generate basic information on young women in order to strengthen capacity building activities and to develop appropriate programmes, besides collecting information on various indicators for programme monitoring. After three years of community-based intervention through multiple approaches across the five districts, this study (endline) has been conducted to assess the effectiveness of the different components of CHARCA intervention, and their impact on five core issues addressed through different sets of programmes and activities, namely, awareness, capacity building, improved services, support system and enabling environment. The specific objectives of the CHARCA endline study are:

- to have a comparative analysis with the baseline survey in order to measure changes in terms of knowledge, attitudes, behaviour and practices with respect to women's vulnerability to STIs and HIV among CHARCA sub-populations in the five districts, and
- to evaluate the process adopted by CHARCA intervention in terms of engaging different stakeholders in collective action at state, district and community levels to reduce young women's vulnerability to HIV/AIDS.

The study has been conducted using a combination of quantitative and qualitative tools in all the five districts. It adopted a suitably developed research design to measure the impact of CHARCA intervention by estimating change through tangible behavioural parameters. Sample sizes to capture expected outcomes in some of the key behavioural indicators across the five different districts of CHARCA intervention have been arrived at on the basis of the five factors typically used in surveys with probability samples – the observed value of the indicator in the baseline survey (expected magnitude of change) which can be attributed to the programmatic response rather than due to fluctuation of sampling with the computed sample size, confidence level, statistical power and design effect.

The major issues and findings are based on information collected during the endline survey as well as the panel data, in which some of the married respondents who were part of the baseline study were

---

* The districts are Aizawl (Mizoram), Bellary (Karnataka), Guntur (Andhra Pradesh), Kanpur Rural (Uttar Pradesh), and Kishanganj (Bihar).

re-interviewed to assess the impact of CHARCA intervention under a cohort approach. Major issues that emerged after a comparison with the baseline data are presented briefly, under different sections, highlighting the emerging features that have programmatic implications.

Knowledge of reproductive and sexual health issues in the process of growing up

- Healthcare providers as a source of information on reproductive and sexual health issues to young women during the process of growing up have increased in almost all districts after the baseline survey. Equally important is the contribution of schools and teachers in imparting information on family life education to adolescents during the process of their growing up. Thus, CHARCA programmes and activities have reoriented the flow of information among adolescents in their intervention areas, which has emerged time and again during KIs and FGDs.
- Knowledge of a location of getting male condom by women varies greatly across the five CHARCA districts. There has been a significant increase in the proportion of women in Aizawl and Bellary, who reported medical stores, health personnel and NGOs/ CBOs as major locations/places. The proportion of women who reported health personnel as sources of getting male condom increased in all districts baring Kanpur. On the other hand, NGOs/CBOs as sources are reported by a higher proportion of women in the endline survey in Bellary, Guntur and Aizawl. The panel data also supports increasing knowledge of source of getting a male condom among young women across the CHARCA districts.
- The level of awareness and knowledge about the availability of at least one source of getting male condom has also increased among unmarried women. A relatively larger proportion of women in Guntur, Bellary and Aizawl knew about all the four different locations of getting male condom compared to those in Kanpur and Kishanganj.
- There has been an increase in reporting of menstrual problems in the last 12 months prior to the survey in all the CHARCA districts, especially among those exposed to the media. In case of treatment for menstrual problems, private hospitals/clinics have been the most preferred place. However, the proportion of women visiting government hospitals/clinics for the treatment of menstrual

problems in the last 12 months has increased in all the CHARCA districts, which can be attributed to the efforts made by CHARCA programmes and activities as part of its mandate to improve reproductive and sexual health services.

Awareness and knowledge about reproductive and sexual health

- Awareness about HIV/AIDS has shown tremendous improvement in four of the five districts between the two surveys. A significant increase has also been observed in the level of awareness among young women in the panel sample, which may be attributed to the range of programmes and activities organized by peer educators under the CHARCA intervention. NGOs/CBOs and health professionals have emerged as main sources of information for young women and men in the endline survey.
- The level of awareness about HIV/AIDS among young men and women appears to depend more on social characteristics such as education and exposure to media. However, a significant increase in HIV/AIDS awareness among those exposed to media in all the districts can be attributed to the macro- and micro-level programmes and activities organized under the CHARCA intervention. In fact, the levels of awareness about HIV/AIDS in the CHARCA districts as per the endline survey are much higher than that of NFHS-3 for the respective states, which signifies the impact of CHARCA intervention.
- Effectiveness of the efforts made by CHARCA peer educators in enhancing awareness of HIV/AIDS at the community level is evident from the fact that a considerable proportion of women and men in all CHARCA districts, except Kishanganj, reported getting information on HIV/AIDS from CBOs/NGOs and health professionals. The panel data also supports the contribution of health professionals in enhancing community level awareness of HIV/AIDS.
- More than three-fourths of the young women in each of the five districts and 84–99 per cent of young men perceive that using condom consistently during each sexual intercourse can prevent HIV/AIDS. This reveals the effectiveness of CHARCA programmes, as these estimates are many times higher than those estimated for India as a whole in NFHS-3 (20% among young women and 37% among young men). The change in the perception is also quite significant in the panel sample. More young women aged 13–16, illiterate, unmarried, rural residents, working as labourers and

not exposed to media do not perceive and are less likely to be aware that consistent use of condom during each sexual intercourse can protect a person against HIV. However, the gap in such awareness among young women is found to be wider by exposure to media and education, especially in Kanpur and Kishanganj.

- Compared to the baseline results, each district records a substantial increase in young men's awareness of condom use as protection against STI or HIV/AIDS. The effectiveness of the condom, despite its low use in all the districts, is also expressed strongly by many young men.
- In three of the five districts (viz., Kishanganj, Bellary and Guntur) there has been a substantial increase after the baseline survey in the proportion of young men knowing about other preventive measures, such as 'checking blood prior to transfusion', 'sterilizing needles and syringes for injections', 'avoiding sex with CSW' and 'sex with only one partner', in all the districts, barring Kanpur.
- A drastic decrease in the proportion of young women with at least one misconception about HIV/AIDS in all the districts except Kishanganj is consistent with the extent of increase in awareness over the CHARCA intervention period. However, young women who are more likely to have at least one misconception about acquiring HIV/AIDS than others belong to the age group 21–24, illiterates, non-members of CBOs/NGOs, and those with no exposure to media. Therefore, any community-based intervention should target these groups through innovative approaches reinforcing the messages on a constant basis.
- One-third of the young women in Bellary, 36 per cent in Guntur, 19 per cent in Kanpur, 15 per cent in Aizawl and 8 per cent in Kishanganj have ever been tested for HIV. The pattern of HIV testing in the last 12 months prior to the survey reveals that 18 per cent of young women each in Bellary and Guntur, 11 per cent in Kanpur, 8 per cent in Aizawl and 6 per cent in Kishanganj were tested in the last 12 months. The corresponding figures for young men are 2 per cent in Bellary, 28 per cent in Guntur, 0.3 per cent in Kanpur, 12 per cent in Aizawl and 7 per cent in Kishanganj. The extent of efforts made by CHARCA peer educators is clear when we compare the above figures with the NFHS-3 national estimates of HIV testing among youth in India. NFHS-3 estimates show that 2.6 per cent among women aged 15–24 and 1.2 per cent among young men below age 25 were tested for HIV during the 12 months prior to the survey. Thus, barring young men in Kanpur,

the levels of prevalence of HIV testing among young women as well as young men in the different CHARCA districts reflects the achievements of CHARCA in addressing the issues of stigma and discrimination and overemphasizing the need for testing by motivating people to use IVCTC services which is a priority area in the NACP-III in the country.

- A large proportion of young men and women reported positive attitudes towards people living with HIV/AIDS and these proportions have increased over the last three years. Qualitative insights on attitude towards PLWHA affirm a change in people's attitude to PLWHA with a reduction in stigma and discrimination and a very conducive environment for testing and disclosure of HIV status. Contribution of CHARCA functionaries in improving the quality of life of PLWHA cuts across all the five districts where the major contributions have been reported in developing a network of positive people, opening of drop in centres, arranging for ARTs and testing of CD4 counts and treatment of opportunistic infections.

Reproductive and sexual health and women's rights

- The impact of CHARCA intervention in enhancing awareness among women to their reproductive rights has not emerged significantly. There has been a significant decline in the proportion of women who feel that they are free to exercise their reproductive rights. In fact, these are the cultural issues rooted in the process of socialization and hence any programme of such a short duration may not impact on the value system. That is why, even if a considerable proportion of women are aware of these issues, it is not reflected in their perception and behaviour. However, the proportion of such women has increased in the panel data.
- Across all the districts less than one in five young women does not have the ability to refuse sex, and this inability increases among women of younger age group, low literacy and non-members of CBOs/NGOs. However, there is a significant increase in the proportion of women who perceive that they have the ability to refuse sex. The contribution of young female peer educators and effective functioning of women information centres have been perceived to bring qualitative change among young women.
- The proportion of women who reported forced penetrative sex declined significantly between the two rounds of CHARCA

surveys – the lowest in Aizawl and the highest in Bellary. Similarly, there has been a decrease in reporting that husbands do not respect their decisions about unwillingness to have sex. There is a substantial decrease in the incidence of forced sex in Aizawl, Kishanganj and Guntur. On the other hand, in Kanpur, Guntur and Aizawl, more men reported, in the endline survey, that they respect their wife's decision when she does not want sex. This is a significant improvement over the baseline survey. These findings indicate the reach and penetration of CHARCA programmes among young men and in creating an enabling environment for young women to exercise their reproductive and sexual rights.

- Overall awareness of condom use as protection against STIs/HIV has increased in all the CHARCA districts, but in the last sexual encounter it has declined in three districts. This can be the cohort effect where a majority has not attained their desired family size and most of sexual activity takes place within wedlock. However, the panel data reflects a significant improvement in condom use during last sexual encounter.

Violence against women and support system

- The contribution of CHARCA intervention in reducing violence against women is evident from the programmes and activities of the women information centre, which has not only enhanced the reporting of violence but has been even included in the domain of issues discussed during CBO/NGO meetings. There is ample evidence of women's awareness in the endline survey and collective actions in opposing violence against women which cuts across all the CHARCA districts.
- The proportion of women who needed their husband's permission to visit healthcare services has declined in all districts except Kishanganj. Need for permission to visit natal family has also declined in all districts except Bellary and Kishanganj. The proportion of women who do not need husband's permission to visit neighbourhoods has considerably increased in all districts except in Kishanganj. However, the same for participating in CBO/NGO meetings has declined in all districts except in Bellary. Thus, women's freedom in mobility is very fluid in nature and depends on local and regional culture, tradition and norms.
- The perception that husbands should be accepted even if they have extra-marital relations has declined significantly. However, the difference is not significant between the members and

non-members of CBOs/NGOs. Similarly, the percentage of young women who reported that they do not have ability to refuse sex if they are not willing has declined in all districts. In the endline survey, a significant proportion of women with membership reported that they have the ability to refuse for sex compared to non-members except in Kishanganj.

- Incidence of violence is the highest in Kishanganj followed by Kanpur. Incidence of violence in Kanpur and Bellary increases with age, while in Guntur more young women experienced violence. In Aizawl and Kishanganj, there has been no marked variation in the experience of violence in the last 12 months. Married women in the districts of Kanpur, Kishanganj and Bellary have experienced more violence in comparison to the unmarried women. However, in Guntur, it is the unmarried women who are facing more violence. In Aizawl, both married and unmarried women have suffered the same extent of violence.
- Membership of CBOs/NGOs has a negative relationship with the experience of violence and reporting of violence is lower among women who are members as indicated in Kanpur, Bellary and Guntur. But, on the contrary, violence is higher among women having membership in Kishanganj. Therefore, it is difficult to analyse quantitatively the exact causation of socio-economic and contextual factors on one hand and perception of facing violence itself on the other.
- Sexual violence against women is also the highest among young women in Kanpur, Kishanganj and Bellary. Sexual violence exhibits an inverse relationship with educational attainment in Kanpur, Aizawl and Bellary.
- The proportion of women seeking support, both formal and informal, is highest in Kishanganj, which also marks a slight increase in the case of formal support sought. Moreover, women seeking support from an informal source has shown an overall decline, being highest in Bellary (40%) and about a 10 per cent decline in Guntur, Kanpur and Kishanganj.

Prevalence of STIs and responsiveness of healthcare services

- There has been a decline in STIs in four of the five CHARCA districts that can be attributed to the increase in the capability of young women to identify the syndromes. The decline is higher among the educated and younger women.

- Except in Guntur, young men in the remaining four districts experienced an overall decline in symptomatic prevalence of STIs. The most frequently reported symptoms of STI across the five districts are 'pain during urination' and 'involuntary passing of semen'.
- Utilization of public healthcare facilities among women has increased significantly over the years in all the CHARCA districts, except in Aizawl. This is also supported by an increase in utilization of public healthcare providers for managing STIs in the panel data. However, the utilization of public healthcare facilities for male STIs has declined.
- Perceptions of young women about the quality of care have not changed over the time period. Young women, except in Bellary, report an increase in the availability of drugs in the healthcare centres during the three years' period. In the case of availability of a trained doctor, young women in Kishanganj and Guntur perceive the situation to be better than at the time of the baseline survey. Except Aizawl, Kishanganj is the only district where healthcare components such as counselling, physical examination and follow-up advice are reported to have improved significantly.

Perceived efficacy of CHARCA intervention

- Most young women in all the districts perceive that the intervention of CHARCA has highly enhanced awareness of STIs/HIV/AIDS among people in the project areas. Since assessment of efficacy is based on perceptions, there is a clear difference in the perceived efficacy by education. Women having more than eight years of schooling are more likely to perceive high efficacy of the intervention programme in almost all districts. Women who had exposure to mass media described CHARCA programmes on STIs/HIV/AIDS as highly effective. However, exposure to mass media did not have much impact in Kanpur and Kishanganj.
- Members of CBOs/NGOs perceive the interventions to have high efficacy than non-members. But, in Bellary district, there is no significant difference in the opinions about the perceived efficacy of the programmes between members and non-members. With respect to occupation, most young women who are homemakers consider these interventions highly effective. Also, women working as labourers or in salaried/paid jobs perceive the

efficacy of the intervention to be very high in reducing risk behaviour.

- A majority of men in all the five districts perceive the CHARCA intervention to be moderately efficient in empowering women. A larger proportion of married women having educated husbands consider CHARCA intervention more highly efficient in reducing risk behaviour than those having illiterate husbands.
- Perception regarding the efficacy of CHARCA intervention on different issues has been varying. For instance, a majority of respondents consider that the CHARCA intervention has been efficient in matters related to reducing risk behaviour (as in Aizawl, Guntur and Kishanganj), beneficial to women and in encouraging young women to go for higher education.
- Most respondents also suggest that the intervention has not been very much efficient in improving services and in empowering women to exercise their reproductive and sexual rights.

Strategies to sustain the efforts made by CHARCA in the intervention area

- CHARCA programmes have involved all the government departments concerned with the welfare of youth such as ICDS, PRIs, education, health, etc. Though on a limited scale, CHARCA project activities have been reflected in day-to-day programmes and activities of these departments.
- Village level organizations have been activated and empowered to integrate awareness programmes for a positive change from violence to respect for women in the community and reduction in youth's involvements in different types of risk behaviour including alcoholism and risky sex. There is ample evidence of a reduction in violence against women in the CHARCA intervention areas, though the intensity of the impact has been varying depending upon the effectiveness of the women's resource centres and initiatives of PRIs.
- In most of the schools in the project areas, teachers have been participating in life skill education. Initially there were some problems in organizing such programmes in schools, but CHARCA intervened by organizing a series of parent-teacher interactions which resulted in a very positive change in the school-based awareness programme in terms of life skill education.
- CHARCA has been able to position its peer educators as resource persons in the intervention communities where people often

approach them as a community level contact persons in case of reproductive and sexual health issues and problems. This is a sign of welcome change and provides an opportunity to consolidate the project by greater involvement of peer educators in sustaining community-based efforts for awareness and capacity building of youth with the technical support of outreach workers selected from the same area.

- CHARCA has been able to develop a district level network of positive people and providing different types of support to improve the disclosure of HIV status in order to improve the quality of life. There is an urgent need to synergize a network of positive people and district level IVCTCs so that positive people can continue to get a similar type of support system that CHARCA has been proving during the last couple of years.
- The findings of the endline survey suggest that the basic reason for violence against women is their inferior status in a male-dominated society – educationally, economically, politically and socially. There is evidence that CHARCA has contributed to women's participation in the programmes and activities of WIC and community-based organizations including mahila mandals and self-help groups. Therefore, addressing violence against women should be prioritized as a central issue in all the programmes and activities designed to improve the health status of women in general and reproductive and sexual health in particular.
- In order to reduce gender-based violence, it is essential to bring changes right from the familial environment to the societal norms leading towards attitude and behaviour of people towards the worth of women, and their social security and rights. To address violence against women more effectively, there is need for effective advocacy efforts so that it can be recognized as a larger public health issue and not merely a legal issue.

There is a crisis of support services available for abused women, as well as programmes designed to educate women directly about minimizing their risk for violence and harm. Ending physical and sexual violence requires a long-term commitment and strategies involving all sections of the society. It is important to address domestic violence through educational and sensitization programmes such as community education, education in schools and colleges, educating health and medical practitioners, organizing programmes for the perpetrators and spreading public awareness on violence against women through the media.

Bibliography

Bhende, A. (1994), 'A Study of Sexuality of Adolescent Girls and Boys in Underprivileged Groups in Bombay', *Indian Journal of Social Work*, Vol. LV(4), pp. 557–71.

Dixon-Mueller, R. (1993), 'The Sexuality Connection in Reproductive Health', *Studies in Family Planning*, Vol. 24, No. 5 (September–October, 1993), pp. 269–282.

——. (1993), *Population Policy and Women's Rights: Transforming Reproductive Choice*, New York: Praeger.

Germain, A. and J. Ordway (1989), *Population Control and Women's Health: Balancing the Scales*, New York: International Women's Health Coalition.

Goyal, R. (2005), *Socio-psychological Constructs of Premarital Sex Behaviour among Adolescent Girls in India*, Jaipur: Indian Institute of Health Management Research.

Greene, K., D. Rubin and J. Hale (1995), 'Egocentrism, Message Explicitness, and AIDS Messages Directed Toward Adolescents: An Application of the Theory of Reasoned Action', *Journal of Social Behaviour and Personality*, Vol.10, pp. 547–70.

Harms, G., A. Corea, S. Iyambo, F. Radebe, H. Fehler and R. Ballard (1998), 'Perceptions and Patterns of Reproductive Tract Infections in a Young Rural Population in Namibia', Second European Congress on Tropical Medicine, Liverpool, UK.

International Conference on Population and Development (1994), *Programme of Action* (PoA).

International Institute for Population Sciences (IIPS) and Macro International (2007), *National Family Health Survey (NFHS-3), 2005–06: India: Volume 1,* Mumbai: IIPS.

Jejeebhoy, S. (1998), 'Adolescent Sexual and Reproductive Behaviour: A Review of the Evidence from India', *Social Science and Medicine*, Vol. 46, Number 10, pp. 1275–90.

Khanna, A. and R.S. Goyal (2005), 'A Study of Adolescent Girls in Rajasthan', *Journal of Health Management*, Vol. 7 (1), pp. 91–107

Kishor, S. and K. Johnson (2004), *Profiling Domestic Violence: A Multi-country Study*, Calverton, Maryland: ORC Macro.

Lhungdim, H. and R. Verma (2004), 'Sexual Behaviour of Male Youth in Rural India: A Five-state Study', in T.K. Roy et al. (eds.), *Population, Health and Development in India: Changing Perspectives,* Jaipur and New Delhi: Rawat Publications, pp. 222–40.

Marston, C. and Eleanor King (2006), 'Factors That Shape Young People's Sexual Behaviour: A Systematic Review', *Lancet,* Vol. 368, pp. 1581–86.

McManus, A. and Lipi Dhar (2008), 'Study of Knowledge, Perception and Attitude of Adolescent Girls Towards STIs/HIV, Safer Sex and Sex Education (A Cross-Sectional Survey of Urban Adolescent School Girls in South Delhi, India)', Vol. 8 (12).

National AIDS Control Organization (NACO) (2001), *Knowledge Attitude and Practices of Young Adults (15–24 years): Disaggregated Data from the National Behavioural Surveillance Survey*, New Delhi: National AIDS Control Organization, Ministry of Health and Family Welfare.

Oommen, N. (2000), 'A Decade of Research on Reproductive Tract Infections and Other Gynecological Morbidity in India: What We Know and What We Don't Know', in Ramasubban and Jejeebhoy (eds.), *Women's Reproductive Health in India,* New Delhi: Rawat Publications.

Rasheed, P., A. Khan and M. Zaheer (1978), 'Awareness of Unmarried Girls Regarding Population Problem, Human Reproduction and Family Planning', *Indian Pediatrics*, Vol. 15(9), pp. 735– 45.

Singh, S.K., H. Lhungdim, A. Chattopadhyay and T.K. Roy (2004), *Women's Vulnerability to STI/HIV in India: Findings of the CHARCA Baseline Survey,* Mumbai: International Institute for Population Sciences (IIPS).

Smith, A., P. Agius, S. Dyson, A. Mitchell and M. Pitts (2002), *Secondary Students and Sexual Health* (Summary of Findings from the 3rd National Survey of Australian Secondary Students, HIV/AIDS and Sexual Health).

UNFPA (2004), *Sexually Transmitted Infections: Breaking the Cycle of Transmission*, New York: United Nations Population Fund.

Verma, R. and H. Lhungdim (2002), *Rural Sexual Behaviour in India*, Project Report, Mumbai: IIPS and UNFPA.

——. (2004), 'Sexuality and Sexual Behaviours in Rural India: Evidence from a Five States Study', in Verma, R., P.J Pelto, S.L. Schensul and A. Joshi (eds.), *Sexuality in the Times of AIDS: Contemporary Perspectives from Communities in India,* New Delhi, Thousand Oaks & London: Sage Publications, pp. 156–76.

Verma, R.K., S. Sureendar and M. Guruswamy (1997), 'What do School Children and Teachers in Rural Maharashtra Think of AIDS and Sex', *Health Transition Review,* Vol. 7, pp. 481–86.

Whitt, J.K. (1995), 'Current Research on Children's and Adolescents' HIV/AIDS-related Knowledge, Attitudes and Behaviour', *Journal of Pediatric Psychology*, Vol. 20, pp. 37–40.

WHO, UNICEF and UNAIDS (2002), *Young People and HIV/AIDS: Opportunity in Crisis,* Geneva: WHO/UNICEF/UNAIDS.

World Health Organization (WHO) and Joint United Nations Programme on HIV/AIDS (UNAIDS) (2000), *Guidelines for Second Generation HIV Surveillance.* Geneva: WHO and UNAIDS.

Index